Survivor

A Memoir of Forgiveness

Cynthia Toolin-Wilson, Ph.D.

En Route Books and Media, LLC
St. Louis, MO

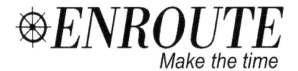

En Route Books and Media, LLC
5705 Rhodes Avenue
St. Louis, MO 63109

Cover credit: Dr. Sebastian Mahfood, OP, with a photo of Ma

Contact us at contactus@enroutebooksandmedia.com

ISBN-13: 978-1-952464-78-2
Library of Congress Control Number: 2021937841

Acknowledgments

I want to express my heartfelt gratitude to my husband, Raymond Charles "Bill" Wilson, for his patient and loving support of me during this lengthy project, and in every aspect of my life. He encouraged me when the writing was not going well and congratulated me when the words flowed easily. He has the purest heart of any man I know.

From the Creative Writing Program at Albertus Magnus College, I want to thank Dr. Paul Robichaud, who served as the Director of my final project and taught me how to edit my own work; Prof. Eric Schoeck, for teaching me how to approach nonfiction writing and particularly memoir writing; Charles Rafferty, for introducing me to the work of many authors; Sarah Wallman, who was a constant source of encouragement during the writing and editing process; and Prof. Robert Hubbard, who taught me about writing as a business and was a constant source of encouragement during the publishing process.

I want to thank my friends who read my manuscript and made editing suggestions (in alphabetical order): Dr. Ronda Chervin, Sherry Lowe, Ann Talaga, Prof. Heather Voccola, and Annette Wilcox.

And I would like to particularly thank my publisher, Dr. Sebastian Mahfood, OP, of En Route Books and Media, for his support and patience.

Author's Note

I write memoir. My art form is unique because I begin the process of writing by selecting life events that reveal the unifying themes of my life. I ignore all the others. Out of potentially millions of events, I focus on only those 20 or 30 that depict me in a range of circumstances at different stages of my life and toss away the rest in the garbage bin of the forgotten. I then try to describe those events as accurately and clearly as possible, but this is difficult given the passage of years and sometimes of decades.

The time factor is important, though, because although it makes the writing difficult, it also makes the writing possible. I can only write about my life as a memoirist, not as an auto-biographer or a novelist, after the seasoning of time and the work of self-reflection. I believe this is because, as I live my life, I cannot see the immediate effect of events on me, nor can I detect a pattern to my behavior. Usually, I cannot see the unifying themes of my life because current events stand in the way of my understanding and blind me to the possibilities of the reality before me.

As a memoirist, I have mulled over the events of my life for more than forty years. Many of these occurred over sixty years ago; some occurred before I was born.

The short version of my memoir is that I am an abortion survivor. In 1949, my mother tried to chemically abort me, and when I was eleven years old, she told me the story of that attempt. For many years afterwards, I reacted to that information by making many of the same mistakes Ma and Pa had made, although to a greater degree. When I engaged in what I now realize was self-destructive behavior, I thought I was being independent, revolutionary, and avant-garde. When I started to look back at that time of my life, however, I could see my behavior seemed as if I had become a mutant hybrid of the worst of Ma and Pa.

In 1988, I converted to Catholicism. Within a few months, I began to understand the marital and familial dynamics between Ma, Pa, and me. The reasons behind Ma's self-abortion attempt became clearer, and I understood many of its consequences on my physical, psychological, spiritual, and social life.

As of February, 2021, I have been Catholic for over 33 years. During those three decades, I learned to listen to my memories, and as I did, I remembered more of them. I tried to understand the reasons behind the actions of others and my slowly evolving reactions to this new information. Slowly, I grew to understand and forgive the three of us, and my deceased husband.

Now I tell my story because I want everyone to find what I have found – the healing power of forgiveness.

Prologue

When I reflect on my life, I always return to the beginning – not to the beginning of my life – my conception or birth, but to the beginning of when I first realized something was seriously wrong in my family. That is where I start my story.

"As soon as I started to bleed, I stopped taking the medicine. I was afraid I might die." As soon as Ma said those words to me, I knew she had just told me she tried to kill me before I was born. I was a few months shy of being twelve years old.

A few minutes earlier, she asked me to sit in the kitchen chair. She said she wanted to talk to me about "something important." I wondered if I had done something wrong, and if so, what it could possibly have been. I thought I was being a good girl, but maybe she thought I had broken one of her many rules. I sat up very straight, pressed my shoulders into the back of the chair, and flattened both of my feet on the floor. I kept my hands still in my lap. I wanted my body posture to let her know I was paying perfect attention to her.

Ma's face was serious, even stern, and her voice didn't sound like it usually did. She started to say something and stopped, then started again. She was hesitating before speaking, as if trying to find the perfect words to convey her thoughts. Beads of sweat lined her upper lip, and I could smell her body, the odor of one not often washed. I thought I must have done something really bad. I spent extra effort trying to look attentive. I lifted my head and tried, unsuccessfully, to make eye contact with her. I really wanted her to know I was giving her my full attention.

While she took her time formulating her thoughts into words, I remembered the last time she made me sit in the same kitchen chair. It happened when we had "the talk" about sex, about the birds and the bees. I was not quite eleven years old.

Ma acted funny that day too, as if she wanted to be in another room instead of standing in front of me and telling me about the facts of life. She told me to be careful or a boy would put himself inside me. I wondered what she meant. I sat still, understanding this was something very serious. Then she added that if that happened, it would hurt and "you won't be a good girl anymore."

When I told her, I didn't know what she meant, she looked aggravated, like I was stupid. She said a boy would try to put his pee-pee into my pee-pee. I thought, "How confusing!" Isn't pee-pee what I do in the toilet? But because she was upset, I nodded as if I understood what she told me. That would appease her, I thought, so I nodded my head again and again like a Bobblehead Doll on steroids.

Unfortunately, I really still did not understand what she

said. Having never seen a naked boy, I had no idea of male anatomy, or of how a boy could put himself inside me. In fact, I didn't know female anatomy either, so I couldn't imagine where a boy would put his pee-pee into me. The conversation with Ma did not enlighten me on the topic.

But the conversation, or perhaps I should say "the monologue," we were about to have was much more serious than the previous one about sex. This one was about death: my death. As I mentioned, I quickly understood that she had tried to kill me before I was born. She continued speaking and her words devastated me. She explained that when she told her father she was going to have a baby, and that she did not want one, he went and got the medicine she needed to make her bleed, to make her "lose" me. Or to speak bluntly, to kill me.

She continued to talk. I felt stunned. I wished she would stop talking long enough for me to understand better the information she had just given me. Ma tried to kill me with medicine. Odd. I thought medicine made you feel better if you were sick. *Why would she try to kill me with something that was intended to make people feel better? Didn't she love me? Would she try to kill me again? Was that the reason she was telling me?*

Within a few minutes of my sitting in that kitchen chair, Ma had told me that both she and Grandpa tried to kill me. I couldn't understand how that was possible. The way Grandpa treated me made me happy. He always paid attention to me, patting me on the shoulder if I had done something well. He gave me gifts for no occasion, but because he thought I would

3

like them. He gave me two hard plastic jointed dolls, a nurse and a soldier, each five inches tall. I was surprised and happy when I saw them. I later found out he probably stole them from the playroom at the Congregational Church where he worked as a janitor. I enjoyed seeing him every day because I loved him, and I thought he loved me. Every time he saw me, he smiled his toothless grin, and the wrinkles in his cheeks became more noticeable.

I found it hard to believe that these two people whom I loved, and whom I thought loved me, had contemplated my murder. I wondered again: *they tried to kill me?*

I thought I should talk to Pa about all this if he came home from work. I refused to believe he would have been involved, and besides, Ma had only mentioned herself and Grandpa. I knew Pa was a drunk and had girlfriends – Ma had informed me of his affairs – but sometimes it seemed like he really cared about me. Once in a while, he would surprise me by giving me a toy he bought at the drugstore, or an old Indian head penny he found at the flea market for my collection. On the other hand, sometimes – well, okay, most of the time - he ignored me. I reasoned that if he had tried to kill me, he wouldn't care about me at all. Certainly, he wouldn't surprise me with little gifts if he didn't love me.

In the following days, weeks, and months, I wondered how much of what Ma told me I should believe. How much could I believe? I started to think about my other family members. Uncle William? Aunt Jody? Ma's relatives who lived in Bristol

– Joan, Louise, Rebecca, Susan. Did they really love me, or were they only pretending to care? Then I wondered about her friends. Christy? Gerrie? The list of potential killers grew in my mind, but I never thought Pa was one of them.

Ma's cousin Joan especially came to my mind. Her husband was a devout Roman Catholic. She was neither devout nor Catholic. When Joan married her fiancé Frank, she promised the priest that when they had children, every one of them would be baptized Catholic. Ma and Pa's entire family was not Catholic. In general, we were afraid of Catholics and did not understand what they believed, other than that they wanted to convert everyone and obeyed the Pope. Pa would talk about the men he worked with, saying, "He is okay – but he is Catholic." His comment implicitly said everything that needed to be said: *be careful, don't trust him, he is Catholic.*

Joan loved Frank enough to lie to the priest. She had no intention of having children who would become part of the Catholic Army of the Faithful. Her parents had warned her to be careful of Catholics. They told her the Knights of Columbus, the handsome men that marched in the annual Independence Day parade, didn't carry swords for ceremonial reasons. The Knights carried swords to rip open the bellies of pregnant women who were not Catholic. They would do this once the war between Catholics and everyone else broke out. Lying to a priest was an acceptable thing to do in her mind. He might be an important man in that army, an archenemy. Why was there such hatred and fear of the Knights of Columbus? I assume it was because they wore uniforms like soldiers and carried swords like soldiers. But they were not soldiers – they were Catholics. I think people thought the uniforms and weapons revealed that the Knights were preparing to fight the enemy. And their enemy would have been all non-Catholics.

Ma told me one time that Joan had a potion she drank every month to make sure she didn't get pregnant. She added that if Joan ever did get pregnant, the baby would "go away." Joan never did get pregnant, or if she did, the baby "went away." I don't think her husband Frank ever knew about the potion and probably thought one of them was infertile. When Ma told me this, I initially didn't believe that such a potion existed. I have since found out that there are chemicals that can be taken very early in pregnancy to cause an abortion; if they are taken every month, they act as a contraceptive.[1]

Joan died of ovarian cancer when she was in her fifties. When I think of her, I wonder if the potion caused her disease and death. But more often, I wonder if she helped Ma either make the decision to try to kill me or provided her with the name of the medicine that she needed to cause an abortion. Ma could then have given that information to Grandpa before his trip to the drugstore.

Joan had no moral problem in preventing pregnancy without her husband's knowledge or in deceiving the man she loved during their entire marriage. She knew how to do it effectively,

---

[1] An excellent source for this type of information is online at sisterzeus.com.

so why wouldn't she help Ma abort a baby Ma didn't want?

I think about Grandpa on that day. He had to walk down Burnham Street, turn left on Dexter Street, and turn right on Cranston Street, to get to his friend's drugstore. He must have known he would have the abortifacient because the druggist was somewhat of a shady character. He sold liquor from his back room on Sundays when the blue laws were still in force in Rhode Island. I can only wonder what other services he provided to his customers.

Grandpa walked all the way to the drugstore and all the way back. It must have taken him over an hour to walk both ways, go in the drugstore, make small talk with the druggist, and buy the abortifacient. I wonder what he thought about – something as insignificant as sports scores or the latest news he read about in the newspaper? Or something more important, like the death of his only grandchild? Did he wonder if his daughter would survive the medicine, or if the medicine would cause the unborn child to suffer? Did he hesitate to think that he could raise the child if his daughter delivered it instead of killed it? I wonder how quickly he walked. Quickly, so that the deed would be done? Slowly, so he could consider alternatives? I think of the beat of his steps on the sidewalk and wonder if they may have mimicked my heartbeat.

Did Ma wait anxiously at the bay window, waiting for her father to come back with the medicine? Was she relieved when she saw he was holding a brown paper bag in his hand as he walked up the two flights of stairs to the front door? Did she hesitate before drinking the liquid?

Meanwhile, I was deep inside her womb, doing what embryos do – growing, thriving, living. I imagine if she hadn't taken the medicine, I would have been normal. But she did, and I am not.

When I sat down in the kitchen chair that day, I loved Ma and Grandpa, and all their relatives and friends. I was happy. When she got through telling me that story, my feelings for her left me the same way the light leaves a room when someone turns off the power switch. I started to engage in conspiracy theory. I wondered then and I wonder now, *who else was involved in trying to kill me?* That question plagued me for decades.

When Ma was finished talking, I stood up and simply said "Okay," and left the room.

But I was anything but "Okay" for the decades that followed, until at age 38, I discovered the healing power of forgiveness.

Chapter 1

The House on Burnham Street

To write memoir about my early life, I have to describe the house on Burnham Street in Providence, Rhode Island.

Ma and Pa bought the century-old duplex on Burnham Street years before I was born. As a child, I could see it was not well kept, but it had one claim to fame: it had been a speakeasy in the 1920s. As I did not know what a speakeasy was, Pa explained that it was a secret place where people could buy drinks when drinking alcohol was illegal. A man would stand at the entrance and when people knocked, he would open a sliding window in the door. If the people who wanted to enter whispered the correct password to him, he would open the door for them. I decided the man who had that job had to be responsible and strong.

The idea of living in a house that once was a speakeasy fascinated me. Over time, I imagined people dressed in their best clothes: men in hats and suits, and women in dresses and high heels with matching pocketbooks, carefully going down the three cement stairs to our cellar. I could picture them sitting at round tables, sipping Gin Rickeys or Sidecars in sweating glasses, gossiping and flirting while they smoked Lucky Strikes or Modianos. They would get up to dance the Charleston, Jitterbug, or Lindy Hop until they tired, and then return to the tables to continue socializing.

I remember comparing the dark damp cellar of the 1950s with its past imagined glory of the 1920s. The comparison depressed me. What had once been a place that I pictured as filled with people having a good time was now just a dirty old cellar.

In the 1950s, the cellar contained a round, black, coal furnace near the dusty coal bin. The furnace looked like an oversized robot, with its arm-like pipes and a door that opened like a mouth hungry for coal. The delivery man must have used a cellar window to get the coal into the bin, adding to the thick coat of back dust. Eventually, Pa converted the coal furnace to a natural gas one. Along the wall, Pa hung shelves made from lumber left over from one of his projects. The shelves were full of Pa's tools, canning jars, and comic book collection. Although part of the cellar floor was cement, most of which was cracked or crumbling, much of it was dirt. When I was older and looked around the cellar, I could see there had never been room for round tables or dancing. I suspected people didn't come to the speakeasy to have a fun evening but to buy a bottle of moonshine or homemade wine. I understood that it could easily be a speakeasy, though, because the windows were so high that they were above Pa's head. I realized that no policeman would be able to see into the cellar, so the illegal alcohol sales could go on unnoticed.

What I remember most about that house, apart from my fascination with its speakeasy history, are the heating, the plumbing, and the sleeping arrangements. The layout of the house on Burnham Street is still clear to me. Ma and Pa renovated the duplex into a one-family house before I was born. The two central staircases remained, but the petition between them was largely removed. We lived primarily on one side of the house, and in the winter, we just occupied the kitchen and living room on the first floor. To keep the cold out of the part of the house heated by the gas range, Ma reduced the living space by closing off the right side of the house and the stairway to the second floor with heavy curtains.

The two sides were almost identical. Each had a kitchen, living room, and bathroom on the first floor, and bedrooms on the second. The bathrooms were small, with only a toilet and sink. The house was built without any bathing facilities.

I imagine that when I was very young and the house was heated with coal, it must have been warm. But when Pa converted the furnace to natural gas, Ma said she was afraid of the possibility of a gas explosion or fire, so she turned the furnace permanently off. That was at least partially my fault.

I was about ten or eleven years old when Ma's Aunt Jody was babysitting me. The gas furnace was new, and I saw the thermostat as a toy. I played with it, pushing the dial way up to turn the furnace on, and then way down to turn the furnace off. After about five or six rapid changes in temperature, the furnace's safety mechanism kicked in and turned the furnace off completely. Jody, who was an exceptionally nervous woman, called the gas company emergency line. A gas repairman came to the house and thoroughly checked the furnace for any problems. He was still there when Ma got home. She thought there was something seriously wrong with the furnace although the repairman explained that there was nothing wrong with it.

Neither Jody nor Ma believed him.

As a result of my childish fun, we never had heat in that house again. I never told Ma or Pa, or Jody, the truth. For one thing, I was terrified of my parents and their anger. Better to be cold, I thought, than make them angry. I also thought Ma would eventually come to her senses and turn the heat on, or that Pa would make her keep the house warm in the winter, but neither of those things ever happened. I remember many winters when the house was so cold that there was ice on the inside of the windowpanes.

The kitchen and bathroom on both sides of the house had water. My parents must have turned the water off in the winter on the side of the house we wouldn't be inhabiting. When it was cold, the faucets in the kitchen and bathroom always had to be dripping or running, so the pipes wouldn't freeze. And the cabinet doors in front of the kitchen sink had to be left open, so some heat could reach them. The house had no hot water during any season, and the only heat in winter came from the gas stove in the kitchen. To wash dishes or to take a sponge bath, Ma heated water in a tea kettle on the stove and poured it into either the kitchen sink for dishes or the bathroom sink for sponge baths. Ma also kept a pan of water on the stove, so the two rooms we lived in all winter – the kitchen and living room – were moist and somewhat warm.

We didn't have a bathtub until I was about ten years old. Pa increased the size of one bathroom by reducing the size of the kitchen. He added a bathtub. He connected the tub to the drain but not to the other plumbing. This meant we couldn't take baths because there was no way to get water into the tub. That didn't much matter because we had no hot water. Once or twice a year, Ma would heat big pans of water on the stove and pour them into the bathtub. She would adjust the water temperature by adding cold water. I would sit in two or three inches of water to bathe. I remember thinking it was a wonderful luxury! I never wanted to get out of the bath. I wished I could have bathed all day every day. I never saw either Ma or Pa take a bath in the tub. They both preferred the occasional sponge bath in the bathroom sink.

Washing our hair was also a major production. This was done in the bathroom sink. Ma had to heat a lot of water on the kitchen stove so we could wash our hair and then rinse it. I usually washed my hair in the late spring and early fall, twice a year, every year. We used bars of Ivory soap, not shampoo.

I have a picture of me posing in Roger Williams Park. The main thing that stands out in that black and white photo is my hair. Since I was not wearing a coat in the picture, it must have been early summer. My hair was so filthy it was stringy.

If the photo was taken in June, I wouldn't wash my hair again until September or October. I cannot imagine what it would have looked like by then.

We used the same sink to clean our teeth, too. I don't remember Ma or Pa owning a toothbrush. Both had some teeth when I was young. Pa had a few, but they were stained and filthy, with big gaps between them where other teeth had been. Ma eventually had no teeth; I suspect they rotted in her mouth. She kept going to the dentist, and each time she came home yet another tooth had been pulled. The last time she went she had had so much Novocain over the years that she had a reaction to it. I did have a toothbrush and toothpaste, which I rarely used. Pa told me I didn't have to use either because it was just as effective to wet your finger and put baking soda on it, rub it on your teeth, and then rinse out your mouth with handfuls of water.

That bathroom sink saw a lot of action. On occasion, we took a sponge bath in it, and about twice a year, washed our hair in it. Pa shaved in it. I brushed my teeth in it. We sometimes washed clothes in it. Yet, I do not recall the sink ever being washed between uses by any of us. I remember, when I was young, taking my fingernail and scraping grayish-black crud out of the basin of the sink for fun, wiping it on toilet tissue, and throwing it in the garbage.

The first two showers that I took are burned in my

memory.

When I was a teenager, I got to take a shower and wash my hair with shampoo on two different occasions. The first time was when I went for a sleepover in Warwick, RI, with the granddaughter of one of Ma's friends. I was probably 13 or 14 and was invited there for her birthday party, which was near St. Patrick's Day. For her party, she had a birthday cake with green frosting and green ice cream. I can never have a pistachio ice cream cone without thinking of that visit. When I woke up in the morning, I took the first shower of my life, and washed my hair with shampoo. I couldn't believe what a luxury this was, to use shampoo, and to have warm water cascading over my body. I thought, this must be what a mermaid feels like every day.

The next time I showered was during a sleepover at Ma's Uncle Sherman's house in Connecticut when I was 16 or 17 years old. Ma loved this uncle. He impressed her with what she thought was his lifestyle and with the fact that he seemed successful. I think she was envious, or perhaps even jealous, of him. He had a home, a nice car, and an "important" job as a factory supervisor. He asked Ma if I could go on a short vacation to the house where he, his wife Marla, and his adult stepson lived. Ma said I could, so we left that afternoon in his car. He treated me nicely, explaining about toll booths and why we would take one road rather than another. He talked to me as if I were an adult, and he made me feel important. Perhaps more importantly, he made me feel noticed.

When we arrived at the house, Marla served lunch, and then Uncle Sherman took me into his darkroom to take black and white photos of me sitting on a stool. When he was done, he turned off the lights and let me watch as he developed the pictures. He explained exactly what he did in each step of the process. He gave some of them to me. When I look at those pictures now, I realize Uncle Sherman had instructed me to sit in seductive, almost provocative poses. He had me sit on the stool with my back and shoulder straight, pull my stomach in to try to touch my backbone, and take a deep breath. Now I realize that pose made me more attractive to him. He had me put one foot on a lower rung of the stool than the other, which exposed more of my legs. He took pictures of me facing him and from the sides.

After the photo shoot, Uncle Sherman and Marla took me for a ride to a five-and-dime store. Uncle Sherman bought me a plaster Buddha statue. We returned to his house, and I got ready for bed. I took a shower and washed my hair. My reaction was the same as the first time I had showered. Warm water and shampoo! I knew I could have taken that shower for as long as I wanted. It was heaven. I just could not believe the delicious luxury of a shower.

But that shower came at a price. Later that evening I went to bed in the guest bedroom. It was a beautiful room, in my mind, like a room in what I considered a fancy magazine, *Family Circle*. It had clean sheets, a soft pillow, blankets, and a bedspread. The furniture all matched. I could not believe how lucky I was to have this little vacation. I thought I understood why Ma loved her Uncle Sherman – he was kind, generous, and successful.

After Marla turned out the lights, Sherman came to see me. The room was dark, so it took me a few seconds to realize that he was standing at the side of the bed. I had not heard him walk in, but I must have seen some movement to realize he was there. He was fully clothed, and softly said to me, "See what you've done to me." He didn't say it as if it was a question, but a statement. Uncle Sherman took my right hand and put it on what I now know was his arousal. At the time, I was too naïve to know this was a sexual act, or inappropriate, or abusive. He stood there for a minute or so with my hand on him, as if he expected me to do something. As an adult, I realize what he expected me to do. But as a child, I had no such knowledge. Then he whispered, "You just want me to lose everything." As he turned away, my hand fell back to the bed. I saw him walk out of the room because my eyes were now accustomed to the dark. I rolled over and went to sleep.

The little vacation, the shower, the Buddha, all came at a price. But I grew in wisdom because of that incident. I now know Uncle Sherman was a loser. Yes, he owned a small ranch house and was married to a woman who kept it nicely decorated and clean. But he was also a great uncle who tried to seduce his great-niece, and then blamed her for his actions. I hesitate to accuse any man of being a pervert, but I think he was one. And I think I was not the only girl he tried to abuse. He probably would have gone further with me if no one else had been in the house. I think the only thing that stopped him was his fear of the consequences.

When I look at those pictures, I am disgusted. Uncle Sherman was the first adult who paid attention to me and made me feel important. He made me feel special. But the entire vacation was about him and his attempt to seduce me. When I look at those seductive pictures, and I think he probably kept the most enticing ones, I assume he must have gone into his darkroom, looked at them, and pleased himself.

On the ride home, Uncle Sherman acted like nothing had happened. He talked about the history of the towns as he drove through them. When we arrived at the house on Burnham Street, he said he hoped I had had a nice trip. He gave me a brand new five-dollar bill to spend on anything I wanted. Then we went into the house, and he and Ma talked for a while before he left. He bent over and kissed me on the cheek. I remember his face had the soft, wrinkled skin of an old man, and I could smell his aftershave - Old Spice or Clubman I think. I wonder if that is why, when I started to date, I preferred to be with men who didn't use scent.

I did not speak to Uncle Sherman for years. I think he may have been embarrassed by his actions, or more likely, afraid that I had told my mother about his behavior. I saw him when he came to Providence for his brother's funeral, but I avoided him. I saw him after I married and was pregnant. That time, he took my husband and me for a ride in his car, acting like a sophisticated and suave man. I knew that his appearance and behavior was a sham. A few years later, I saw him when I went to his funeral. I was happy that he was contained in the casket and would soon be buried under six feet of earth. I fantasized that his casket should be wrapped with chains and locks so that he could never escape, as if he were a vampire. And in hindsight he was that – a vampire whose abuse of young girls would keep him alive and young in his mind.

I think I loved showers because I knew Ma, Pa, and I were dirty people with minimal personal hygiene. We were filthy. The story of my toy kitchen hints at this fact. When I was very young, I had a pink toy kitchen. It had a tiny stove, sink, and refrigerator, with a mirror over the sink – all in one unit – maybe 12 inches long. One day, I got a boil on the right top of my forehead. It looked really gross. Ma took me to Dr. Rivas by cab, to see what was causing this thing to grow on me. He told her it was a boil and to have me hold hot compresses on it. It was angry looking, red, and swollen to the point of shininess. I didn't go to school because I felt embarrassed to have this thing, that would soon be as prominent as a unicorn's horn, growing out of my forehead. A few days later, I was sitting at the kitchen table, playing with my toy kitchen, and looking in the mirror, when the boil broke. Unbelievable rot. The shiny red boil that was so visible on my forehead, split in the middle and lumpy yellow pus combined with strands of blood slowly oozed out of it towards my eye. I still wonder if it came from being dirty.

The fact that I was filthy – that we were filthy – rose to my conscious thought, but I had once believed I looked cute. It wasn't that the thought "I am cute" crossed my mind; it was just my mindless state of being. I had no reason not to think I was so. I thought I had nice clothes and hair, just like the other girls in grammar school. I did not, but I couldn't see any difference between us. I had toys, maybe even more than some of the other kids. Yet, I never received an invitation to other girls' houses, and I never invited them to mine. The reason was simple. I was hideously ugly and just plain filthy. I stunk, as my clothes probably did. My head was too small for my body. I had buck teeth that a chimpanzee would have been proud of, and my teeth were black from lack of attention. My left eye wandered. I was stoop-shouldered. I washed my hair a couple of times a year. And I had a really weird gait.

I look back and understand why the other kids didn't want to be friends with me. A few years ago, when I came across the picture of me in Roger Williams Park, I felt shocked at my appearance. I wondered why no one ever called the police or child protective services.

The last thing I remember from the house on Burnham Street was the sleeping arrangements. As a small child, I slept in a bedroom with gut-wrenching scary wallpaper. It had a light pink background, with a pattern of Little Miss Muffet and the spider that sat down beside her. On the wallpaper, the spider was huge and black, and considering the repeats of the pattern, there were hundreds of them in my room. I believe that wallpaper is why, to this day, I am unreasonably afraid of spiders. Or, more honestly, I am gut-wrenchingly terrified of them, big or small.

When I grew a few years older, Ma moved me to another bedroom with blonde furniture and a lamp that had a blue and gold shade. When I turned it on at night, the shade looked like a blueish purple sky with gold rain. I loved that bedroom because it was such an improvement over where I had slept before and because I thought Ma must have really loved me to buy the furniture for me.

In the summer, Ma and Pa each had a bedroom. I never remember my parents sleeping together. On many occasions, Ma slept with me in my new bedroom, or in the spider room, instead of her own room. Pa's bedroom fascinated me. His room contained a bed with a colorful hand-knit afghan on it, an oak desk, and a lawyer's banister (a cabinet, that is, with lots of shelves) filled with books by Zane Grey, Arthur Conan Doyle, and Jack London. The desk and bookcase fascinated me the most, as if in the finest life I could imagine I could have such a room and read anything I wanted at any time.

Pa didn't use his bedroom to sleep. Instead, he took a piece of plywood, put it over the stairwell, put a mattress on it, and built a small barrier on the edge so he wouldn't roll off the bed and fall down the stairs in a drunken stupor. That is where he slept in the summer. He used his coat for a pillow, sleeping on the mattress, with blankets but no sheets.

I loved Pa's area over the stairwell. It seemed like a play-room to me. I could sit on his mattress, look out the tiny window at the entire backyard, and hide in the hall closet. The area was like a passageway to a dream world. I would hide in the closet, pull the one-panel curtain across the opening, stand perfectly still, and imagine what I would do with my life, where I would live, what I would achieve. I loved that little closet. I always felt safe there, but I wished it had a door so I would be safer.

I feel sad when I think about my childhood dreams, and that I only felt free to think of them when I sat alone on a piece of plywood over the stairwell. I never shared my dreams because I was afraid of being belittled and being the source of humor. I hoped to be a brilliant writer, live in North Dakota, and be at best a plain-looking woman.

In the winter, I slept on a canvas cot in the kitchen in front of the stove, which had a pot of water simmering on it all the time. Ma slept on a couch in the living room. It was the kind of sleeper couch that folded down, so the back of the couch became half of the "bed." Pa had his partition in the front hall and the small bedroom he had made for himself behind it.

I believe it is because of these sleeping experiences that I can still sleep anywhere, in any position, or situation, with or without bedding. I can sleep sitting in a kitchen chair, perfectly still. But I truly prefer to sleep on a couch. I feel safest on a couch, or to be more accurate, I feel less vulnerable. I put my back against the couch back and really press myself into it. Then I put all the covers over my head, as if I am a hibernating bear. I have mastered holding a corner of the covers up with my hand while I sleep so I can breathe.

I reason that if I sleep on a couch, a person could only get to me from the front, and I would probably see him coming. But since I am under the covers, I might not even be seen. When I am alone, I will sleep on a bed, although it seems like an undeserved luxury. Even in a bed, I bury myself completely under the covers so that if anyone approaches, I might be mistaken for what looks like an unmade bed. When I vacation, I prefer to be in a camper. In a camper, I can still sleep on the couch, but in a hotel, I have no choice but to sleep in a bed.

A few years ago, I watched a crime show on television and in it, a wealthy and mentally ill criminal slept on the closet floor in his luxury apartment. I thought, what a great idea! Unlike the criminal, I could have a complete wardrobe and many boxes in the closet. If I slept on the closet floor, no one would see me because I would be beneath the clothes and behind the boxes. I have never actually slept like that, but I must admit it had great appeal.

Apart from the plumbing and heating issues, the house on Burnham Street could have been a beautiful home. In the backyard there were three trees: a big maple, a small maple that Pa called "Cynthia's tree" (or Cyndi's Tree). I wondered if Pa planted it when I was born. There was a cigar tree that grew between the other two. There were two unpruned pink rambling rose bushes and several hostas. Pa had planted English Ivy, Hollyhocks, Tiger Lilies, and Four O'Clocks. Ma had a row of tulips that came up every spring. She said they "stood up like tiny toy soldiers at attention." On the right side of the yard was a long row of lilac bushes. They bloomed beautifully in the spring, and I think that is why I like flowers with many petals – lilacs, geraniums, and hyacinths.

Pa built a beautiful cement patio in the backyard. The three of us had watched a TV movie that depicted what would happen if there was ever an atomic bomb strike. Within a week of watching it, Pa was out in the backyard digging a hole. He dug from the painted brick foundation out towards the trees, maybe a little less than half the width of the house. Ma thought he was building a bomb shelter to protect his family, but he was really building a patio.

It is not surprising that Ma thought this. In addition to the TV movie, children in school at that time were being taught to hide under the desk in case the area was hit by an atomic bomb. Good grief! Were adults so naïve that they didn't know about the fire, the radiation, or the broken glass and collapsing buildings from an atomic bomb? I have thought of that patio and our school instructions many times, but especially after Pa and I watched *The Day After* as a grown adult in 1983.

The Burnham Street house could have been beautiful. It was a nine-room home, with the local history of having had a speakeasy in the cellar. It had gas heat and two bathrooms that could have been modernized to include bathing facilities. There was off street parking that would have required a brave driver to risk going in and out of the narrow uphill driveway. There were trees, flowering bushes, and some flower beds in the backyard. People could have sat outside in the summer on the back patio and enjoyed the sun or shade, depending on the time of day. There could even have been a barbecue.

Yes, the house could have been beautiful, and the family within it could have been happy. But neither became a reality.

The house was on a small hill, with two flights of stairs leading to the front door, which was flanked by two bay windows. The average person walking by the house, if they gave it a second thought, would probably have thought it nice and that a happy, or at least normal, family lived within it. The house wasn't nice, although it could have been with some updating and maintenance. And the family was not happy, or normal, by any definition I have ever seen.

The best way I can describe the house is by comparing it to the Munster Mansion at 1313 Mockingbird Lane. Although Ma and Pa's house was not as large as the Munster Mansion, it stood tall on that hill. It had many windows, and the architectural angles were similar. But the real similarity, the weirdness, was not the physical building itself, but life within the house. The Munster family was composed of the father,

Herman, a Frankenstein lookalike; the mother Lily, and her father Grandpa, both vampires; the son, Eddie, a werewolf, and Marilyn, a normal-looking niece. For all their freakishness and weird exploits, and with all the issues they had to deal with – like what to feed vampires and a werewolf for dinner – the one advantage the Munsters had over my family was that the members of that family loved each other. They were a real family, and the members cared about each other. But in my family, only weirdness could be seen in the void where there should have been love.

Chapter 2

Personal Relations on Burnham Street, Part 1

Why was the house on Burnham Street such a terrible place to live? The first issue was control. Ma controlled the house with her fear that the natural gas furnace would explode. She refused to turn the furnace on even during the coldest days of winter, resulting in a constant lack of heat and hot water. But Pa controlled the money. He worked in a gold-plating factory as a foreman, but Ma didn't work after both she and Pa gave up modeling for the Rhode Island School of Design over thirty years before.

As was common in the 1950s and 1960s, Ma stayed home and kept a clean house by daily dusting and vacuuming. She must have cooked because neither she nor I starved to death. She cared for me by making sure I stayed alive, and she occupied me with toys so I wouldn't interrupt her soap operas. Her priority during those days was cleaning the house, smoking Viceroys, and watching soap operas. At night, she smoked Viceroys and drank. She was unhappy with her life, and I think that made her a mean drunk.

But Pa was meaner. I think Pa let Ma control the house because then she would leave him alone. But he controlled her with his money and his adultery. On many Sundays, Pa would heat water on the gas range and pour it into the bathroom sink. When he was finished shaving, he would look at Ma and say, "I'm going out for a while." He would walk out with a swagger, leaving the stink of cheap aftershave lingering in the air like a toxic fume. When I was young, I didn't understand why Ma would look so devastated every time he said that. But now I understand what he was really saying: "I just shaved so my girlfriend will like the way I look. I'm going out for a while to be with her." I witnessed the scene more times than I care to count.

The second reason was the meanness. Ma and Pa were mean to each other. They were always fighting. I can't say who started the fights: Pa leaving to be with another woman or Ma screaming about him taking her away from her home in Bristol to live a life of misery. Even if they weren't fighting, a tense atmosphere always permeated the house. Living there was like sitting in a room with a stink bomb and waiting for it to go off.

As an adult, I cannot understand these dynamics. Pa basically told Ma he was going out to meet a strange woman, and she just let him go. In most marriages, both people want to be with each other. I wonder if Ma was mean because she was constantly frustrated and angry, knowing that her husband wanted to be with other women but not with her. And Pa let her know he had many female companions.

Although they were both mean to me, Ma treated me worse than Pa did. They both forced me to take unnecessary medicine. Once a week, on Friday, Pa made me chew an ex-lax tablet. As if that wasn't bad enough, he also made me take a teaspoonful of cod liver oil "to give me a good physic." To this day I will go hungry before I will eat cod. Ma made me take a red square asthma pill that I had to hold under my tongue for five minutes every night, even though I was breathing well.

One night, I was sitting on my canvas cot in front of the kitchen range with the pill under my tongue, getting ready to go to sleep, when Pa came home drunk with a few jazz records he had bought. He said I'd like them. Ma told him I didn't like his music. He stood there and broke every one of them in front of me while he looked me straight in the eye. My heart was breaking. I wanted to say something to Pa, to tell him that what Ma said wasn't true. But I was afraid of what Ma would do to me if I opened my mouth to speak to Pa and the pill fell on the floor.

As I got into my teens, I had a difficult time going to school. I knew I was kind of freaky looking, and by then I realized I didn't wear the same kind of clothes as everyone else. I had a navy-blue dress with a huge Kelly-green bow that hung down past my waist. Even though it made me look like a wrapped birthday present, I had to wear it to school. One year for winter, Ma took an old coat of hers and made it smaller for me. It was made with fake fur fabric in a leopard print with huge black buttons. There wasn't a single girl in school who wore a dress or a coat like mine. Not one. Not even the fat old math teacher with sagging underarms that swung when she wrote on the blackboard had clothes like mine.

One day Pa got angry when I complained to them about my clothes. Pa was starting to shave in the bathroom sink, Ma and I were in the kitchen, and I anticipated Pa's usual ritual. He would say he was going out for a while, and she would act devastated. I decided right then – I have no idea what made me think this was a good idea – that this would be the time to voice my opinion of my clothes. I said, "No one in school has a coat like the one Ma made me." Pa said – "There. I was waiting for you to say something like that. I've watched the other kids, and they have all kinds of coats."

That might have been true. Many girls had heavy wool coats or leather jackets. But how many had a leopard print coat of fake fur? One. Me.

This exchange was an odd experience for me. For one thing, Pa defended Ma's resizing of the coat, even though he knew wearing the coat made me feel ridiculous. I realized Ma and Pa must have been talking about getting a coat for me or deciding what they were going to do to get a coat for me. Ma needed the money for the house, and Pa needed the money for his women. It really freaked me out – they talked to each other about me, but neither one of them bothered talking to me. And then these two people, who never agreed on anything, had sided against me. What interested me further is that on this occasion, Pa just went out without saying a word. And Ma looked victorious instead of devastated. She held her head just a little higher than usual as she struck a match to her cigarette with her nicotine-stained fingers.

Good Times

Not every day in the family was bad. One July 4, when I was eleven or twelve, Ma and Pa took me out to celebrate the holiday. They did not take me out together, but separately. Pa took me to Rocky Point Park in the morning. It was so early that there was little traffic on the road as Pa drove to the Narragansett Bay side of Warwick, and very few people had entered the park when we arrived. When I think back to that day, I suspect he wanted to get this outing over with so he could enjoy the rest of his day with one of his female friends. We walked around, and I rode the merry-go-round and played a few carnival games.

I remember thinking I liked having all of Pa's attention. But we couldn't really communicate. I didn't really know him, or Ma for that matter. And I realized that they did not know me either. I watched them interact, but little of that interaction happened with me, and what did was not positive. I realized for the first time that I had little in common with either Ma or Pa. I didn't know how to talk to adults, and the only things I really wanted to know were why we lived the way we did and why Ma was always so unhappy and mean. Pa would have gotten angry with me if I had asked those questions that resided in the forefront of my mind. I knew he would not answer me, and I also assumed that he would take me home and end our outing.

But there was more going on inside of me than the fear of getting him angry. I didn't understand it then although I later figured out that our connection was nothing more than that Pa and Ma were really nothing more to me than genetic parents.

After Pa drove me home and "went out for a while," Ma took me to my first movie by taxi. I had never been in a movie theater, and I really enjoyed it. We went to see a Disney animated movie. I think it was Cinderella. It amazed me that people could pay for a ticket and go into a theater to enjoy a movie anytime they wanted to have fun. Such luxury! I remember looking around the theater and being in awe of its sheer size – it was the largest room I had ever been in. I stared at its heavy red curtains and the banks of comfortable chairs that were seemingly on a hill. At the time, I thought this must be the kind of building where a Disney princess like Cinderella would live. I wondered, *Why can't I be a princess and have a beautiful room like this? One without spider wallpaper.*

After the movie, Ma took me to Luke's Chinese restaurant in downtown Providence, RI. It was my first time in a restaurant. We had chow mein sandwiches and chicken chop suey. To this day I remember how I loved that chow mein sandwich – chow mein piled high on a warm hamburger bun, with crunchy Chinese noodles. It was the most exquisite food I had ever eaten. Ma sat across from me at a table for two, but we ate the meal in silence.

Once again, I was struck by the lack of connection and my inability to communicate with either Ma or Pa. I never saw Ma outside of the house unless she took a taxi to a doctor's office, or to Uncle William and Aunt Jody's tenement, ten houses from where we lived. And here Ma and I were "enjoying" part of a day together.

I've thought about that day many times and wondered what was going on in their lives that both of them chose to spend a half day with me, entertaining me and giving me new experiences. Although I enjoyed the day, it made me sad at the same time that the two of them didn't spend the whole day with each other and with me.

I saw this as another example of them talking to each other about me, but neither of them to me. We never conversed much among the three of us, and I lived in an almost nonverbal environment. Perhaps the silence I lived in is why I can't hold up my end in a conversation. I am socially inept, and blunt. I say what is on my mind in a sentence or two, and then I don't say anything. And I usually eat my meals in silence.

As an adult, I have had people tell me that I am conceited and feel superior to others. They say I treat people with disdain. But in my heart, I know it is because I don't have the skill to converse on mundane matters. I just don't know how to make small talk like everyone else.

On another July 4, Ma took me to Bristol, RI, for the annual town extravaganza. Her cousin Joan's husband, Frank, picked us up in their car and brought us to Joan's parent's house. Susan and Jack, Joan's parents, lived over a shop and had a patio that was the roof of a second attached shop. All the family would go out on the patio to watch the parade. I had never seen a parade, and I was very excited. I don't know where Pa was at the time, but Ma was having a wonderful time, talking with relatives, eating chorizo and peppers with tomato sauce, laughing and smiling, standing at the railing.

When the Grand Marshal of the parade, a man Ma had gone to grammar school with, marched by the house, he looked up, saw Ma, and gave her a smile and a wave of recognition. She kept repeating, "He remembered me! He remembered me!" Her voice was joyful and filled with a longing that even I could recognize. I never heard her voice sound like that before or after the day of the parade. The sound of longing in her voice made me sad for her; it almost made me pity her. It was as if she knew her life would have been better if she had not left Bristol and married Pa. I thought of the monologue when Ma told me she tried to abort me, and I think I understood her situation in 1949 better than I had before.

I don't know if Ma and the Grand Marshal had been romantically involved when they were young, but I am sure she would have preferred to be with him rather than Pa. I doubt they ever dated because he was of Portuguese descent. In the early 1900s, there would have been strong social mores against their dating, both because of ethnicity and religion. I assume he was Roman Catholic.

It was an odd experience for me. Clearly Ma knew I was sitting in front of her on the roof porch. But it was as if she couldn't see me, nor recognize that I was observing her. I felt like a ghost, present but no more than a transparent being who might be seen or not. It made me sad because it was the happiest I ever saw Ma. A man from her past remembered her, and she reacted with complete joy. When I think back to that day, I realize Ma must have had an insufferably miserable life, full of regrets.

I remember there were other good times. She decorated the house for Halloween and Thanksgiving every year. I have always loved those holidays, and I wonder if it was because she cared enough about me to make the house look festive. To this day, I decorate my house for the fall holidays, starting immediately after Labor Day. Summer is gone. I get out the oranges, golds, and rusts of fall, and welcome the harvest. I bring out my pumpkins and gourds, pilgrims and turkeys, much as Ma did over half a century ago.

The fall is my favorite time of year. But when I remember celebrating the fall holidays in the house on Burnham Street, I must define them as odd. Ma would make up Trick-or-Treat bags, and I would hand them out at the door. I do not remember going out Trick-or-Treating, but I do remember having at least one Halloween costume, or at least I remember the polyester fabric in the costume – although I do not remember what it was supposed to disguise me as – a witch or a princess, I suppose. I think I might have handed out candy dressed up in that costume. I also know I had Halloween candy of my own, but I don't remember how I got it. I suspect the adult neighbors brought it to me, or it was left over from what Ma bought.

For Thanksgiving, there was always a feast of eggnog, turkey, bread stuffing, mashed potatoes, turnip, gravy, and two kinds of canned cranberry sauce, jellied and whole. The three of us would eat together on elegant Depression Glass plates. We sat together as if we were a real family. For dessert, we would have Duncan Hines spice cake with vanilla frosting, and Ma would make whole dates stuffed with peanut butter and rolled in confectionary sugar, and peanut butter fudge. I love those delicious foods, but I don't eat them anymore because they make me so sad. I want to cry because of the lost opportunity to be a family.

After dinner, Pa would leave, Ma would do the dishes, and I would watch the rest of the Macy's Thanksgiving Day Parade on TV.

On occasion the three of us would take a ride to Shun Pike, a place outside of Providence where Ma and Pa owned a long, narrow lot of land with a rundown shack on it. The three of us would have picnics there with Ma's Bristol relatives, and I would try, unsuccessfully, to play with my cousins who were closest to my age. Again, it seemed, my lack of communication skills interfered with the development of possible relationships.

The most positive thing Ma ever did for me was to teach me how to read. When first grade ended, I could not read well enough to go into second grade. The principal of my school came to the house unannounced. He and Ma sat in the living room, with me as an odd onlooker. He talked to Ma and told her he would let me pass from first grade to second grade if she taught me how to read that summer. He glanced over at me with a look of pity, then back at her with a stern face. I don't know if he thought I was too mentally challenged to learn how to read or if he didn't think she would follow through and teach me. Or both. To her credit, she did teach me. Every afternoon, between lunch and the beginning of her soap operas, we sat on the couch together and she taught me how to read.

Learning how to read opened up the world of information to me. It took me a while to understand how to do it, but eventually, I was able to research topics of interest to me. Soon afterwards, I discovered that I could find relationships between different topics and go more deeply into topics of interest. Almost three decades later, that skill led to a fine graduate education. When I earned my doctorate in sociology at the University of Massachusetts at Amherst, I thanked Ma on the acknowledgments page of my dissertation for teaching me how to read. I am not sure what her reaction would have been if she had read it – pride, happiness, jealousy, disinterest? I don't think these feelings are mutually exclusive, so she might have had them simultaneously. I will never know because she died the year before I graduated.

Back to Everyday Affairs

When I was a young girl, I couldn't see or interpret the dynamics of Ma and Pa's relationship. When I was in my teens, Ma told me the story of how they met. She was in her early twenties, and Pa was in his late teens. Ma fell in love with him, as he was quite the rakish rogue when he was young. Pa would put on a suit and walk up and down the street so people could admire him. He wore his hat at a jaunty angle. He was handsome, and he had a devil-may-care attitude that women found irresistible.

Ma also told me that within a year of their marriage, Pa was cheating on her. One of his girlfriends told Ma that Pa preferred to sleep with her because Ma didn't move in bed. Ma looked at me when she told me this, and said, "I was a young girl. I didn't know I was supposed to move." It was pathetic to hear her voice as she said she didn't know how to make love. It was a cross between sadness and regret for lost opportunities with the man she had loved. Although I did not know what she meant, I thought, *"Remember to move when you sleep with a man."* She never got over that conversation with one of Pa's women. I think it permanently broke her heart. She had given herself to Pa, and he had let her know that he found her inadequate.

Nor did she ever get over the multitude of betrayals that occurred after the first one. Pa was a serial adulterer. He never gave her a chance to forgive him. For him, there was always another woman, or two, or ten, to seduce, to have sex with, and to leave.

Pa hid his affairs from everyone except Ma and me. I am sure every woman who fell victim to his seduction thought she was the only woman he had ever looked at or ever desired. He was a talented seducer, a flatterer. Ma told me that when they started dating Pa called her his Little Pansy Face and said she had ears like beautiful seashells.

Ma was one of those silly women who was easily seduced by Pa, and once she figured out that she was not special, but just another conquest, she never forgave him. She never forgot the difference between what he said to her when they were first together and how he treated her after he married her. She proved that the old saying, "Hell hath no fury like a woman scorned" was rock solid true. And until the day she died, Pa and I felt that fury.

I think Pa at least made a cursory effort at being a parent, although he didn't have a lot of patience. One time, Pa took me to the grocery store, the Star Market. I was excited to be involved in the adult activity of grocery shopping. When we came back home, I was helping carry the groceries in when I dropped one of the full brown paper bags. I tried to save the bag, but in the process, I twisted my right ankle. I limped up the stairs and sat on one of the top steps, crying. I remember being in agony, and Pa was nice to me. He put his arm around me, and I said my ankle burned. He explained that nothing in the grocery bag I had dropped would burn me.

Then he realized a glass bottle of bleach had broken and the bleach had gone over my foot. I remember he half carried me as I hopped into the living room to lay on Ma's couch where she slept at night. For the next two weeks, I lay on the couch, and if Dusty the cat tried to jump on the couch, I screamed in fear that he would land on my ankle. Pa could not tolerate my screaming and yelled at me. I don't think he understood that I screamed in anticipation of additional pain.

Two weeks passed and they never took me to the doctor.

That poor ankle. When I was a teenager, a friend accidentally slammed a car door on it.

And then when I was in my fifties, I tripped on a shoe and sprained the same ankle again. The initial injury had made that foot weak.

I never thought much about that first ankle injury until, when I was 60 years old, I fell down a flight of cement stairs on vacation. My husband took me to the Emergency Room, and the staff took x-rays of the ankle. They told me I had a sprain and to follow up with my primary care physician. When I returned to Connecticut, I made an appointment with my doctor, bringing with me a disk of the x-rays from the Emergency Room. He looked at the x-rays on the disk and said, "Oh, that's the old broken ankle, right there." I thought, "*The old broken ankle? Like from when I was a kid and no one took me to the doctor? When I twisted my ankle on the stairs? That broken ankle?*"

When I found out that my ankle had actually been broken when I was young, I went home and cried. It broke my heart. All I could think of was me, as a little girl, hurt and needing help, but not receiving any. My needs were ignored by Ma and Pa, their friends and family, and neighbors. Didn't Ma and Pa care about me at all? I was a filthy little girl, with dirty hair and teeth that were stained black, and I had a broken ankle. Didn't anyone see that I was in trouble? Why didn't anyone call the authorities?

Chapter 3

Personal Relations on Burnham Street, Part 2

I remember Ma and Pa talking at that old Formica kitchen table with metal legs, drinking quart bottles of Narragansett beer. I don't know what they talked about when they drank because I was sleeping on my canvas cot in front of the gas range. I know it was winter because we were living in only two rooms.

The beer came in brown bottles, and when they took the metal caps off and the yeasty aroma entered the room, I thought the beer stank. I never developed a taste for beer and have drunk only the equivalent of two six-packs in my life. I think beer tastes like Pa's dirty undershirts smelled.

Every week, Pa brought cases of Narragansett Beer into the house, and on occasion bottles of beer in paper bags. Ma and Pa liked to drink, and when I was young, they liked to drink together. I think that other than screaming at each other, their favorite thing to do was to drink together. Eventually Pa graduated from beer to wine. Ma would sometimes drink a deep red wine in what looked to me like juice glasses, which were brought from Italy by her friend Teresa. The glasses had frosty etchings of grapes on them, and Ma would drink from them, full to the brim with wine. She remained a beer drinker for years, but stopped drinking in her 50s, sometime before Pa did.

I was happy when Ma stopped drinking because she was just plain mean when she drank. I would be reading or playing and for no reason that I could discern, she would suddenly say, "You'd better be careful. There are crazy people in your family!" She implied that I carried crazy genes inside of me, just waiting to attack. I often wondered, since Ma and I were related, why she didn't realize that meant she carried the same crazy genes she thought I had?

I thought that if she stopped drinking, she would stop saying such mean things.

But I was happy for nothing. Ma didn't stop being mean when she stopped drinking. As she got older, she actually got meaner. I once read of a woman who became saddened when her mother stopped drinking. She had always assumed her mother was a mean drunk, but when her mother stopped drinking, she realized her mother was just mean. That would describe my mother. Ma was just rattlesnake mean, a miserable bitch.

Pa continued drinking for a few more years after Ma stopped. He graduated to glasses of wine and eventually to gallon jugs of white wine that cost a couple of dollars. Pa drank so much that his pores stank of rancid wine. And, as is often the case with drinkers, Pa lied.

When I was about twelve years old, Pa told me that when I was ready to go to college, the money would be there for me. I wouldn't have to worry about paying for school. Silly me, I believed him. I felt such excitement. I would be the first person in the family to graduate from high school, and then I would go to college. When I graduated from Central High School, I filled out college applications for every school that interested me. I dreamed of being in a sorority in Boston or attending a big state university where I would learn wonderful things. I would leave Providence and never come back.

I gained acceptance at several colleges. When I told Pa I had been accepted and was ready to go to college, the money wasn't there. Either he never had it, or he drank it all away, or he spent it on his women. I was heartbroken. I learned the true meaning of betrayal. And why was I surprised? Pa had betrayed Ma for years. Why wouldn't he betray me? He had lied to her for years. Why wouldn't he lie to me?

Perhaps one of the weirdest dynamics in that house was Ma's fear of thunder. Ma was terrified of thunder and lightning. Something must have happened to her when she was young to make her so afraid of storms. In grammar school, I had to write a report on thunderstorms, so I borrowed a book from the school library to learn about them. It was an old green clothbound children's reference book with a drawing of lightning on the cover. "How could you bring a book like that into the house when you know I'm afraid of thunderstorms?" she screamed at me. I couldn't understand how she could be so upset by a drawing of lightning on the cover of a book, and it wasn't even a realistic drawing at that.

She was home alone with me one day when a bad thunderstorm struck. I remember the sky became dark, and the wind was gusting. Rain fell sideways. Even I could see that as thunderstorms go, this was a bad one. She got us both into the corner of the living room, as far away from the bay windows as possible. Every time it thundered, she would jump, and her shoulders and upper body would shrink back and to the left. Her face scrunched up in fear. I could smell the sweat oozing out of her filthy pores, the smell of stale sweat. I am still surprised that she didn't place me between her and the windows. I think if there had been a god of thunder and lightning, she would have sacrificed me to him so that she could live.

It seemed that every time Pa and I interacted, Ma got mad. She was jealous of me. I have no idea why. I was not one of his women.

Ma and I did a puzzle on a card table in the living room, and Pa came in just about when we were done. As Pa walked across the floor I said, "Pa, I want you to have the honor of putting the last piece in the puzzle," and I handed it to him. He laughed and put it where it belonged. Ma sat there and I could feel the anger radiating out of her. I think she wanted to let me know she expected me to care more for her than for him. I thought, "No problem there, Ma, I care for both of you about the same. Which is to say, not much."

One day a sample of upholstery fabric came in the mail and Ma said I could have it. I had a little doll that had no clothes, so I thought I would make her a dress from the fabric. I sat at the table and while I was trying to figure out how to make it, Pa came in and asked what I was trying to do. I told him, and he said, "No problem." He took a pencil and traced the outline of the doll's body on the fabric, and then he cut out the pattern. The dress was too small, and the fabric was wasted. I felt sad about that, but Ma was furious. She looked at me with flashing eyes and told me I should have asked her how to make the dress because she knew about sewing. I thought, *"Really? How was I supposed to know that? Did you ever tell me? Did you ever sew in front of me?"* Now I know that the problem was that Pa didn't include a seam allowance when he cut the fabric.

Probably the most important positive presence in my life at that time was Ma's father, Grandpa Herb. Like everyone else in that house, he was an alcoholic, but he was a happy drunk, not a mean one like Ma and Pa. He was a happy-go-lucky man, who had been a house painter in Bristol, Rhode Island. His claim to fame was being part of the crew that painted the Mt. Hope Bridge. He had no fear of heights and would paint the highest uprights of the bridge. Sometimes, to show how fearless he was, he would do headstands on the top of those highest uprights. That seemed to be his way of goofing off from work. I have some worn old photos, faded brown with age, of Grandpa Herb doing a headstand on an upright of that bridge. At some point, he had fallen while on the bridge and landed on his back. I don't know how serious the injury was – this happened long before I was born – but I know his back bothered him for the rest of his life.

Ma loved him. I could see her love for him, and I couldn't understand why she didn't feel that way about me. I loved him too. Grandpa Herb was just a loveable guy. Or anyway, I loved him until Ma told me, when I was eleven years old, that it was Grandpa Herb who got her the 'medicine' to kill me.

Grandpa Herb lived on Burnham Street with us. He slept upstairs on the side of the house that we didn't use. This must have been when Pa still heated with coal and the house was warm. He would have frozen to death up there in the winter if Pa had already changed the furnace.

I was about 7 or 8 years old when Grandpa Herb started to have serious back pain and began to go to Dr. Rivas. He diagnosed Grandpa as having cancer, but I don't think he told Grandpa that it was cancer or that it was terminal. It took him a while to die. He was so weak, he had to sit on the stairs to get down them one by one. Once Dr. Rivas came and gave him a pain shot. It wasn't too long after that that Grandpa died. In those days, they didn't have anything but painkillers to help cancer patients.

I remember the morning he died. Ma and I were asleep in the same room. I remember waking up to the sound of Pa yelling for Ma, running up the stairs. "Bud, Bud (he called her), he's gone." Ma jumped out of bed and started to cry. She wailed, "Oh no, now the only person who cared for me is gone!"

After the funeral, which I was not allowed to attend, I asked Ma if Grandpa Herb knew he was going to die. She said she thought so, but she wasn't sure. She had found a piece of paper he had folded again and again, until it was thick. She did not say it, but I think she was trying to tell me he was nervous or worried about dying and folded the paper because of that. I thought he might have folded the paper because he was bored, but I was smart enough not to say that to Ma. I can't imagine that a man dying of cancer wouldn't have had some sense that he was not going to live.

I don't remember Grandma Deb, his wife, because she died when I was two years old. I have heard wonderful stories about her. Like Grandpa, she lived with us. She liked to sit in the hedge-enclosed garden on Burnham Street and read. I love to read and write. We had something in common. We could have been friends. When I found out that she liked that garden, I used to go sit in it and pretend she was there. I missed her even though I never knew her.

Grandma Deb died of a heart attack. When the chest pain started, she screamed for help, but by the time Pa got to her, she was gone. Many years later, Pa said he had a story to tell me because no one was still alive who could be hurt by my knowing it. I got really nervous because I thought it might be another abortion story and I thought if it was, I would die on the spot.

Pa told me Grandma Deb had screamed out one word, "Quick!" And he ran to her. She had a liquid medicine that would bring her back from one of her "spells." So, he ran to the medicine cabinet to get the blue bottle of medicine, opened it, and put it under her nose, hoping it would bring her back. I thought, *"Pa, the dead don't breathe, so it couldn't 'bring her back.'"* He said he smelled the medicine to see if it was still strong. I thought to myself that that was a bad idea. If it was strong medicine for her and he had a good heart, wouldn't it have killed him or at least made him sick? He discovered that she had put cologne in the bottle. She must have used all the medicine and rather than throw the pretty blue bottle out, she used it for a different purpose, as a cologne container.

I could see how sad he felt that he couldn't save her. Maybe he thought that if he had realized the bottle contained cologne, he would have found another bottle of the medicine and still saved her. He seemed to really care about her. When she died, she was much younger than I am now.

Both my grandfather and grandmother relied on the charity of Ma and Pa to take them in when they were old.

As far as I could tell, Pa liked his father-in-law and mother-in-law. Ma, on the other hand, could not stand Pa's father, mother, or his second wife. I am not sure if Ma even went to the funeral of Pa's mother, who died in Kansas City when I was about eight but was buried in Boston. Pa told me that once he had asked Ma if she would take in his parents – meaning, his father and Christy, his second wife – and Ma said no, she wouldn't have them in her house.

While all these things were happening to the elderly relatives, Ma continued to ignore me. She taught me to amuse myself, I believe, so she wouldn't have to interact with me. She would sit me at the kitchen table and give me a toy, and I would play with it for hours. My toys were my babysitters. Eventually, she taught me some crafts, and those became my new babysitters.

While Ma's Uncle William was in the VA hospital, dying of liver cancer, Barbie and Ken dolls became popular.

I told Ma I would love to have them, and she bought them for what I think was my eleventh birthday. William couldn't understand why a big girl like me would want those two dolls. Ma's only concern was if Ken was anatomically correct. When I saw Ken's "anatomical correctness", I wondered what all the hoopla was about the differences between boys and girls.

I had many toys: a metal roller coaster, Ferris wheel, and merry-go-round, an ambulance, a metal dollhouse, dolls with outfits (including shoes), games, and puzzles. Once Pa asked where my toy lantern was, and I said I didn't have one. He said,

"You don't have a lantern? Oh, you have to have one." He said it with such sympathy, like not having the lantern meant I would never find fulfillment as a human being. They bought me a red one, and I remember being confused as to why this new toy didn't bring me the ultimate happiness Pa had implied it would.

They gave me a lot of toys. But it wasn't out of love; it was so I wouldn't bother them. It served me well though because it made me self-reliant and comfortable with being alone. My isolation resulted in my creativity and imagination, and my ability to see relationships between things that others miss. I think, *"Thanks Ma and Pa. You both did me a favor, even if it wasn't what you were trying to do."*

I had two toys I loved more than anything in the world: a metal dollhouse and a set of plastic doll furniture so tiny that I kept it in an ashtray. Pa gave them both away. The dollhouse went to another dirty little girl in the neighborhood who had fewer toys than me. I asked where my dollhouse was one day, and Pa told me he had given it away. Then Ma's Aunt Jen came to visit with her daughter Maria and her two granddaughters, Patty and Pam. Pa gave the granddaughters my plastic doll furniture. I felt a sense of painful helplessness when Pa gave away my beloved things. He had all the power, and I had none. Within a few months, Ma decided to throw out some magazines I had stored in my metal desk. My reaction to her was not the same. This caused a deep sense of betrayal. I knew that she valued the things she had; it bothered me that she did not value my things, even if they were a pile of magazines.

As an adult, I saw a dollhouse that was almost identical to the one my father gave away. When I discovered it on eBay, I bought the two-story metal beauty with a green roof. On the first floor, there is a kitchen, a living room, a breezeway, and a rec room. On the second floor, above the kitchen and living room, there is a nursery, a bathroom, and a bedroom. When it arrived, I was surprised at how small it was, but of course, I was little when I had the original, so it seemed larger to me then.

I still own that dollhouse, and I actually hate it. In some way I think I expected the dollhouse to give me some peace about my childhood. I thought I would be able to look at it, and the adorable plastic furniture, and be deceived into thinking it had been a gift given in love.

Perhaps the loss of the dollhouse and the tiny dollhouse furniture I kept in the ashtray is why I am always decorating and redecorating, arranging, and rearranging my home. I have done pine country, Victorian mahogany and cherry, World War I oak, and modern ebony. Today, my house is decorated in an eclectic style that I call primitive urban ethnic. I am never satisfied, though, with the look I attain when the decorating is complete. I think my houses are where I have lived, but they are not my home.

Another way that Ma taught me how to amuse myself was through crafts. She first taught me how to knit. Ma used to make knit hats that were supposed to look like mink. They didn't; they looked like knit hats made of fake mink yarn in fake mink colors. They looked like what a poor person who had never seen a real mink hat thought mink hats would look like. If a real mink saw their hats, it would roll over laughing at what a human thought a mink looked like.

I remember pestering her to teach me how to knit. One afternoon Ma sat me down on a kitchen chair and handed me two white plastic knitting needles and a ball of ratty looking pink yarn. She cast on and showed me how to make the stitches. I spent the better part of the afternoon busily working on my project. My Grandfather Herb walked through the kitchen and looked at the knitting as he passed by; an hour later he walked by and looked at it again. "Bud," he said to my mother, "why isn't that knitting getting any longer?" She came back and looked at it. "You're not doing it the way I showed you. You're not doing it right." I discarded the knitting and got up to watch what I think was the Mickey Mouse show with Annette and the gang, all of whom I figured could knit better than me.

I was in my 20s before I picked up knitting needles again. I made three afghans and a lion toy, and then I retired the knitting needles forever.

Ma sat me down, again in the kitchen chair. I thought, "*I hate this chair. Every time I sit in it, I either learn something I wish I hadn't learned, or something bad happens to me.*" This time, Ma had bought me two stamped cross-stitch pillowcases, an embroidery hoop, and some embroidery floss and needles. I decided to do some serious work. I am sad to say that the results were not good. My finished project was not something anyone would want to sleep on. My stitches measured at least half an inch long, I didn't cross the Xs in the same direction, and my Xs never met in the corners.

On my own, I decided to make an embroidered picture of a house. I used black floss and drew the picture in my mind: walls, roof, two floors, windows, and smoke coming out of two chimneys. I made the smoke go in opposite directions. I guess there was a new kind of wind that worked from the center line of the roof and blew in two directions. I got bored and made straight stitches between half an inch and one inch long to finish the project. I thought I was being quite creative by using only black thread; other, less imaginative girls, might have used different colors.

In the end, Ma's attempt to keep me busy interested me in handcrafts. As an adult, I became a master crocheter, punch-needle rug hooker, and Victorian crazy quilter. If she had known I would love crafts as an adult, she probably would not have used them to keep me quiet.

I think Ma felt jealous of Pa because he left the house every day and had a life apart from both of us. And I think she was jealous of me because she could see that I was still trying to have a relationship with Pa, or at least some kind of connection.

Sometimes Pa would be at lunch on a weekend. Ma knew he liked sliced cucumbers in vinegar with pepper on them. One day, I took one of his cucumbers out of the bowl. Ma got angry and yelled at me. She said, "Those are your father's," with a tone of outrage in her voice. Since they were in the middle of the table, I thought they were for anyone to eat. I had never had a cucumber fixed this way before, so I wanted to try one. Pa said I could have one, so I did, but I could see the furious expression on Ma's face. I think Ma was angry that Pa was kind to me. And I think she scolded me because she wanted him to think she cared more for him than for me. I thought, *"Gees, Ma, we both know that you care more about the cat than me."*

Chapter 4

Life on Burnham Street After Pa

In the early 1960s, Pa left Ma. He left the house he had bought, the garden he had tended, the wife he had wronged. And he left me.

I have no idea why it took him so long to leave. Ma berated Pa, and her anger towards him was palpable; she yelled at him every time she had the opportunity. I understand why she hated him, but I do not understand why, in light of her constant abuse of him, he stayed even loosely attached to her.

Perhaps he left because he lost his job. Pa was a metal worker, a gold plater. For many years he had worked for the same prominent company, and eventually he worked his way up to being a supervisor, or as he called it, a foreman. Then he was fired. The reason the company gave was that he was stealing. Pa swore he didn't do it. He said his manager framed him, and that his manager had accused Pa of theft to protect himself. Pa threatened to run his manager over with his car and kill him.

Even if it was true that Pa had not stolen the gold, I doubt that anyone would have believed his story. By that time, he had deteriorated from a handsome man into a smelly wino with threadbare clothes. Since he didn't wash himself, I don't think he washed his clothes either. I have seen homeless men on the street who looked – and smelled – better than he. Who would believe such a man?

Pa sat on the same kitchen chair I had sat on when Ma told me about the birds and the bees, and when she told me she tried to abort me. He sat there for weeks, crying, and threatening to kill himself.

Ma and I always thought he stole the gold, as did Dr. Rivas, the family physician, who was a friend of one of the company owners. Ma had been to see the doctor, and while she was there Dr. Rivas had asked her where Pa hid all the gold. He had heard the story of the theft. Ma delighted in telling Pa that the doctor believed he was the thief.

I didn't really care one way or the other if Pa stole the gold, but when I heard the news that Dr. Rivas thought he had, and I knew Ma thought he had, I believed it too. After all, Dr. Rivas was a physician, educated, wore a suit, and didn't smell. Why would I think Pa was telling the truth given the "evidence"?

One day, about forty years later, I was talking to one of Ma's cousins who had worked for the same factory as Pa. I said something to him about how Pa deserved to be fired for stealing. He looked at me, clearly confused, and said, "I don't know how it could have been his fault." It had never, not even once, occurred to me that Pa could have been innocent. I had assumed that when a person is accused of doing something seriously wrong, it is almost certain that the person is guilty.

I suppose to a great extent I had also based my belief of his guilt on his overall moral life. Even when I was a young teenager, Pa's lack of shame embarrassed me. He had a lot of women, and not only was he not discreet about them, he acted proud of his seducing capabilities. If he would commit adultery openly, I reasoned, why wouldn't he steal?

What I do understand is, if I was accused of stealing and I was innocent, and my spouse believed I was guilty, I would either leave him or ask him to leave. That might be what finally made Pa leave Ma and me.

When Pa left, I didn't feel any sense of loss because I saw him almost as much as when he lived in the house. Eventually another company hired him in the same industry for the same kind of work. He kept that job until he became disabled in his fifties.

All the years they were apart, Pa came by every week to give Ma money to run the house. I don't know the amount, but it couldn't have been much because she kept a few bills and some change on the stairs, and she always counted it like she was worried that there wasn't enough. Pa would give her the money; she would figure out what bills to pay and how much to put aside for groceries, and then she would give those amounts back to him to run the errands. After his errands, he would return to the house, shave in the all-purpose bathroom sink, get all duded up and leave. Ma used to say he was going to see one of his girlfriends and to the best of my knowledge, she was right.

One time Pa gave her the weekly money, and when she gave him money to pay the bills, he didn't do it. A few weeks later, I overheard Ma on the phone explaining to the bill collectors why the bills weren't paid. She told them she gave Pa the money, but he had clearly not paid the bills. I could hear the anxiety in her voice; I felt ashamed to hear her practically begging the person on the other end of the line to believe her. When Pa came by the house the next time, Ma and Pa had a fight about it. In the end, Pa just said, "The bills will be paid." After he left, Ma told me that she thought he had given the money that we needed to live on to one of his girlfriends. I think she might have been right, but I couldn't help but wonder if he needed it to pay for an abortion.

After that incident, I thought more deeply about the situation in the house. I realized the problem was that Pa controlled the money. I hated Pa for the money issue, and I hated Ma for being so dependent. I vowed never to let a man control the money, and to make sure that I could take care of myself. I have tried to live by those rules since I left home although it took me a long time to get to a solid level of security.

All the time that they lived apart in Providence, I can remember Ma saying that by living alone, someday she would be free of him. I did not understand what she meant. I think in her mind, if not in the law, she thought that after ten years of not cohabiting with him she could go to court and be free. Then Pa had congestive heart failure and moved back into the house. Her physician, Dr. Rivas, who treated her for emphysema and arthritis, told her that as long as Pa lived in the house, the law would assume they were cohabiting. I can remember the disappointment on Ma's face; she looked dejected and said, "I'll just have to start over." I think she meant in marking the time. Financially, she couldn't have made it on her own, but Ma, I came to realize over time, was really not smart enough to know that.

But figuring out what was wrong in the house, or trying to understand relationships in the house, did not improve matters. I got sick and was not well cared for; Ma got hurt and sick, and she did not receive care; and Pa, who was behind many of the problems in the house, got sick and hurt and yet got care from Ma and me.

Just before I turned 13, I experienced terrible stomach pains. Pa was at the house, and on his way out the door. I told both Ma and Pa I was really sick and needed to go to the doctor. Pa laughed like I was making it up. I said something like, "No, really, I'm sick." He said okay, we would see how I felt in the morning. He left anyway. I told Ma that I really needed to see the doctor, that something was wrong with my stomach. She said, "Fine, if you are so sick, go call the doctor." So, I called Dr. Rivas, and since doctors still made house calls then, he came to the house. Once he examined my stomach, he told Ma I had to go to the hospital.

When Dr. Rivas left, I heard him tell my mother it was the first time a child had had to call him for help. She acted embarrassed and seemed angry with me because I had caused the embarrassment. She behaved like I had deliberately gotten appendicitis but managed to conceal the symptoms until the next day when the doctor's offices were not open. When I think of that night now, I think, *"Really? How does one cause appendicitis?"*

Ma called Pa and told him about the situation. I don't know what he said, but I do know that when they hung up, she called a cab and we went to the emergency room. What a conversation that must have been. I imagine it went like this:

Pa said, "She isn't sick. I saw her."

Ma answered, "But she is complaining. And Dr. Rivas said I had to take her." Pa continued, "It is a waste of time and money to take her to the hospital." Ma answered, "How will I explain it if she dies before she gets to the hospital?"

Pa finally agreed. He said, "Ok, take her to the emergency room. Call a cab. I'm not driving over there to drive her to the hospital; she has too much imagination."

Pa still didn't believe I was sick. Ma and I took a cab to the hospital. I know now that that is not normal behavior. A little girl, just about 13, in pain and afraid, should not take a cab to the hospital. Ma should have called an ambulance, or Pa should have taken us.

When we arrived at the Emergency Room, the doctor examined me and said I had "a red-hot appendix." That night I had an emergency appendectomy.

From what Ma told me afterwards, the doctor said the appendix looked almost ready to burst. I had no idea then how serious an issue that would have been. I decided that I liked being in the hospital. I wondered if the appendix had burst, would I have been able to stay in that beautiful place longer? Ma gave me attention. Some of her Bristol relatives and her friend Teresa visited me. Teresa brought me a bottle of Jean Nate after-shower lotion. Clearly, she didn't know I did not take showers, so I had no use for the Jean Nate. Because of that gift, I have a special place in my heart for Teresa. She brought me a feminine luxury I had never had and treated me not just as a sick girl in the hospital whom she had to visit because she was Ma's friend, but with respect and kindness.

Pa did not visit.

Ma continued our relationship with Dr. Rivas. A couple of years after the appendectomy, Ma was sitting in a chair near the wall where she had hung two elaborate shadow boxes she had painted glossy red. They were loaded to capacity with chalkware Chinese figurines. With no warning, one box fell off the wall and all the figurines fell on Ma's head. Ma demanded that I call Dr. Rivas. This was the second time that as a child I called the doctor. Dr. Rivas told me to watch Ma in case she had a concussion. I thought, *"Watch her?"* I had no idea what the signs of a concussion would look like, and fortunately she didn't have one. If she had had one, I suppose I would have had to call the doctor again and take care of her out of duty. I thought that would be a terrible inconvenience. I felt very annoyed that I was expected to watch over her when she hadn't even believed that I had appendicitis.

A few years later, Ma went to an appointment with Dr. Rivas. When she came home, she told me he had diagnosed her with emphysema. She told me it was a lung disease, and that she would suffer as if drowning as she died. She thought she had contracted it due to Pa frequently coming home from work covered in asbestos. When she told Pa this, he retaliated against that accusation by telling her he thought that she had contracted it when she smoked Viceroy cigarettes by the carton. I didn't care how she got emphysema, nor did I care that she had it. I could do nothing about her disease and neither could Pa or Ma. She had it, so she had to deal with it.

I know Ma felt like she had no control over her life, so when she believed she could get control over someone else's life, she went for it. One of the cruelest things Ma ever did was to abuse a widow, and unfortunately, I cannot excuse myself for my part in her behavior.

We had neighbors in the building next door who lived in the first-floor apartment. They seemed an odd-looking couple. The woman was very large. I think she weighed around 300 lbs.

She had what in those days we called "milk legs." Her legs were enormous, and it was impossible to see where knees and ankles were located unless she bent one of those joints. She wore loose cotton housedresses. You could have made a tent with the material in one of those dresses, but they fit her fine. Her husband was a tiny man, short and thin, and also much older than she was, or at least he looked that way to me as a young teenager.

Every once in a while, she would have me babysit her young son. He was about two years old.

One day, her usually sparsely furnished place was packed with junk her husband had found somewhere, or perhaps had been given by someone moving, who didn't need as much stuff, or perhaps who didn't have as much room. Bed frames and old chairs with missing legs, an incomplete set of dishes, and some really old books like a set of encyclopedias which held arcane information jammed the space. Talking to a friend on the phone, the wife complained about all the stuff, and said her husband had said he would be able to sell it and make a lot of money. I commented aloud that they would have to pay someone to take all that junk away, and the next thing I heard, she was her telling her friend what I had just said as if it was her own idea. I realized for the first time, that I could make a statement and that others would listen.

Shortly thereafter the wife went into the hospital because of trouble with her legs. Her husband called and asked if I could babysit so he could go see his wife, and I did. While I was there the phone rang, and I answered it. The woman's voice on the other end of the line said angrily, "Who is this?" And I responded just as angrily – "Who is this?" "Okay," the woman said, "I am his wife." I told her I was the babysitter. Then she said that was ok and asked me where her husband was. I didn't know for sure, but I began to figure all husbands were like Pa, and went off to have a good time without their wives.

About a month later, the wife called me, very upset, and said she needed me to babysit.

Her husband had died. I had an important test at school the next day, so I told her I couldn't because I had to study, and she said I could study while I babysat. Ma started screaming in the background, "Tell her no. Learn to stand up for yourself." So, I said, "I can't babysit tonight." She replied, "I won't be able to see my husband again."

I have regretted my part in that conversation with my neighbor, now a widow with a young child, and hideously overweight. I don't know what she meant by the statement, "I won't be able to see my husband again." Was she was referring to planning his funeral or going to his wake? I cannot imagine how she felt.

Decades later, my husband Jimmy died, and I thought of that night and of that conversation with my neighbor. I thought about how I felt when I went to make the arrangements for my husband's funeral and was supported by two dear friends; how I felt when I went to the wake and saw him in his coffin for the first time; how I felt when I walked out of the funeral parlor the day of the funeral knowing I would never see his face again in this life; how I felt when I walked away from the gravesite, leaving his coffin balanced over a hole in the ground, and depending on strangers to bury him.

Ma was wrong to tell me to stand up for myself that night, but I think she seemed proud that I refused that woman my help. As a young teenager, I was discovering that I had the power to say "yes" or "no" to another person's request for help, and that I alone could determine what I would do. At the time, I unfortunately did not know that I was wrong in what I did and that my bad decision would come back to haunt me on March 14, 2006, when my own husband, Jimmy, died.

I later knew that there are times when a woman must stand up for her rights, but on the night that my neighbor's husband died, I was wrong to stand up for myself.

I never spoke to that neighbor again, nor she to me. She moved out of the apartment a short time afterwards. Perhaps she couldn't afford the rent after her husband died.

Ma was an abusive woman, perhaps because she had been abused and neglected by Pa. She abused me verbally and psychologically, and she neglected all but my most basic needs.

Only once did the neglect and psychological abuse turn to physical abuse. I was old enough to leave the house on my own, and I had a car, so I was at least 18 when this happened. Ma was drinking a glass of red wine, acting like her usual mean self. I prepared to leave the house, and she grabbed me from behind and pushed me against the upright piano she kept in what she called the parlor. Her face expressed drunken hatred. She screamed at me about something – probably sex. Ever since I had turned 13, she had clearly been obsessed with my budding sexuality and whether or not I had inherited Pa's sex drive. She always wanted to know if I was a "slut" like he was a "whore-master." I have no idea what I did, or didn't do, to set her anger off that night.

Ma had not taken into account that I was almost an adult, with the strength of youth on my side. She was just a bitter drunk old woman, old before her time. I didn't think about what I did; I just reacted. I took her by the shoulders, turned her around, and slammed her as hard as I could against the same place I had occupied seconds before. I should have said, "How does that feel, you miserable bitch?" But instead I slammed her back into the piano with each word, to emphasize each one "Don't... you... ever... do... that... again!" I left the house and came back later, expecting round two.

We never talked about what happened between us that night. Maybe she had been drunk enough to think she had won the fight, or to forget that it had happened. Although that is unlikely, considering the backache she must have had the next day.

But then, we never talked. As I grew older, we became more and more irrelevant to each other. We ate meals in silence, and I seldom remember eating with her. On rare occasions when she cooked, she would have the radio on. I remember in 1962 she liked a song "Soldier Boy," sung by the Shirelles. Although I knew she liked it, I tried to get her attention one night when it was on. I kept talking and talking and talking while she made a spaghetti sauce to serve over mashed potatoes. She became so angry that I never again tried to get her attention when she was cooking or listening to the radio. At night I would watch the black and white TV alone. I assume she drank while I watched TV. My life was solitary, and I knew she always secretly watched me for sexual impropriety. The sexual impropriety accusations drove me crazy then. And to this day, I resent them. The only good thing about the fact that she would say those things was that she convinced me of her stupidity.

The two staircases that went from the first to the second floor were divided by a wall because the Burnham Street house had been built as a duplex. The stairs on the right were the ones we usually used. As a child, Ma let me use the stairs on the left as a kind of playroom in the summer. I would sit on the stairs and play with my dolls. As I started to get older, I took pictures of female movie stars and scotch-taped them to the walls of the staircase. One day Ma came over to see what I was doing, and I told her I had just put up a new picture. She asked me which one, so I pointed to it and turned my head to Ma to say, "This one," but Ma had started screaming at me because I had put my finger on the private parts of the star. In trying to point to the new picture, my finger, which could as easily have gone to the star's head, neck, or shoulder, apparently landed in the wrong place.

She screamed and screamed and screamed at me, as if I were a pervert, and to boot, apparently a homosexual one. She loudly accused me of wanting sex and screamed that I was just like Pa. To this day, I think Ma lied about where my finger landed.

But that incident was nothing compared to the weirdness of the black hand incident which happened when I was in high school. I always wore skirts and blouses, or dresses, with a slip underneath, to school. One day I came home from school and Ma was in rare form. She had washed one of my slips in the all-purpose bathroom sink. She started screaming at me that she had found the handprint of a black man on it. Though I was still young, I wasn't stupid. I knew that if any man had had his hand on my slip – which I most decidedly knew had not happened – a black man would not leave a black handprint on it, nor would a white man leave a white handprint. I didn't know how to respond to her accusation. Such a weird accusation stunned me, and I couldn't come up with an answer. She might as well have accused me of having sex with an alien on a spaceship. I wondered if I should explain that hand color could not transfer to clothes? Or should I explain that no man had put his hand on my slip? I tried to explain both.

She refused to listen. Not only did she think a black man had had his hand on my slip, and left a black handprint, but she insisted I had been in my slip when this had happened. I thought, *"Good grief. This woman is a stupid idiot."* I kept trying to explain reality to her, but she just kept yelling louder.

In the end, I never convinced her that she had falsely accused me, and she never changed her mind that must be I lying. It was the first time I realized that Ma was a racist, and a stupid one at that.

Chapter 5

Life Continues on Burnham Street Without Pa

I remember Ma had friends and relatives she stayed in at least minimal contact with when we lived on Burnham Street. Over time they died or stopped coming around, possibly because of their advancing age or their discomfort with our lifestyle.

Ma knew Jennine from when she was a young girl in Bristol, RI. They were classmates and stayed in touch by phone. One day, Jennine decided to take me to see *Gone with the Wind* when it was re-released. I had seen it the week before, but Ma said I had to go anyway. Completely bored, I already knew the scenes, characters, and plot. Jennine knew something was wrong and asked me if I had seen it before. I said no because I knew my mother would kill me if I told her the truth. When the show was over, Jennine was going to get a cab, go to a Chinese restaurant to buy takeout, and then continue to our house. I decided to walk home instead. When I got to the house, Ma was furious. She screamed at me that Jennine wouldn't come to the house now because of what I had done.

Confused, I had no idea I was being rude.

They didn't talk by phone for years, and then one day Jennine called to tell Ma she was dying of breast cancer. I never understood that whole situation. I don't know why Ma didn't teach me some basic social skills or explain what I had done wrong; I don't know why she didn't call Jennine and apologize, or better yet, why she didn't have me call Jennine and apologize.

Another of Ma's friends was Hope, a woman who lived next door in a third-floor tenement. Hope gave us a gas refrigerator because she had bought a new one. At the time, we only had an ice box. She also gave me a doll and I played with it constantly. I just loved it. Then Ma said, "Your other dolls are getting jealous because you only play with that one." This really upset me. Not because it would be a great horror film story – *Revenge of the Jealous Dolls* – but because I didn't want to hurt the dolls' feelings.

Ma's Uncle William would stop by every weekday morning for a couple of hours for coffee. He rented a tenement on the same street, and they would talk for hours. Uncle William had been a submariner in the war. His parents had forced him to join the navy because they wanted to "make a man of him" – I suspect now that he was gay. Even though he was usually her only company, Ma complained about his visits because she wanted to get her housework done so she could watch TV – her "shows" as she called them, the soap operas. Uncle William had cancer and as the disease progressed, he would pull dead skin from his hands, peeling it off and dropping it on the floor into a disgusting pile. This drove Ma crazy. He died of liver cancer, and Ma took in his spinster sister, her aunt Jody, when she was released from the mental hospital.

Uncle William was good to me. He used to save all his change; no matter what he bought, he paid for it with bills, and stashed the change away in a jar. When he rolled it, he would give me what wouldn't fit in the rolls, around a dollar or two, but it wasn't like he owed me anything. It was a pure gift. One time, I misunderstood him to say that he was going to give me all the change he had saved. When I said this out loud, he and Ma laughed at me. I always thought that they were not laughing at my silly mistake, rather they were laughing at me. I started to be more cautious when talking around Ma.

Ma's Aunt Jody kept dollar bills rolled up in jars that she hid in her bureau drawers. When she went to the mental hospital about the time that Uncle William died, Ma had to clean out Uncle William and Aunt Jody's tenement - by cab (it was about 10 houses from where we lived) - and in the process, found the money. Ma told their sister, her Aunt Jen, about the money, and she insisted it all be sent to her, as it should be in a bank account earning interest. I remember Aunt Jody's face when she was discharged from the hospital and came to live with us, and Ma told Aunt Jody she had cleaned out the tenement. Jody said, "Did you find the money?" Ma said yes and told her Jen had it. Jody looked devastated. In one day, she was discharged from the hospital, found out she had to live with Ma - no longer in her home, the tenement - her brother Uncle William had died, and she was broke, robbed by her sister.

I felt bad for Aunt Jody, even though she was clearly crazier than Ma. She took Librium, which she hid in the cracks between the floorboards upstairs in Ma's house. Librium comes in bright blue capsules. How could she think they were well hidden between floorboards that were painted dark brown? If Aunt Jody was watching television and a man came on, like President Kennedy, she would sit up attentively because she thought he could see her. And if she didn't own any lipstick, she would wet her finger, put it on the wallpaper, and transfer the color to her mouth. She stopped hiding money in jars and started hiding it in the toes of her shoes.

Aunt Jody had a hard life. She wanted to be a concert pianist, but her father forbade it, reasoning that a single girl in New York City would become promiscuous. So, Aunt Jody obeyed him, even with his ridiculous reasoning and his arbitrary authoritative decision. That is what women did in those days and still do in many parts of the world today. About five years after she moved in with Ma and me, Aunt Jody finally went totally insane and was institutionalized; she died, in my mind, an unhappy woman who never had a happy life.

When Ma moved the stuff from Uncle William and Aunt Jody's tenement to our house, there were four things Ma wanted – two bronze statues and two porcelain ones. She loved them. But Aunt Jen's daughter, Maria, came on the day of Uncle William's funeral and said, "These will go in my house," and took all four of them. It was Ma's turn to be devastated and my turn to be confused. Why hadn't Ma done what she was always telling me to do, "Stand up for yourself"? Why hadn't she just said, "No, you can't have them"?

The other side of her family, all of whom still lived in Bristol, were Ma's cousins, Frank, Joan, Steve, and Rebecca, who would visit her once or twice a year. They rarely came to Providence, but when they did Frank always drove, and after he got into the house, he fell asleep. One time when Rebecca was leaving, she put money in Ma's hand – five or ten dollars. Ma expressed delight, but I felt embarrassed. I wondered if they came because Pa had left. Years later, when Pa was back in the house, I had that same feeling of shame when a charity group from the neighborhood brought us the food needed to make a Thanksgiving dinner.

Ma's cousins were good people, and generous. Rebecca made Ma a pink shawl of yarn – either knit or crocheted. It looked beautiful. Ma kept it wrapped in plastic in a drawer to keep for a special occasion that never came. I don't know whatever happened to it. One year, Aunt Joan gave me pencils with my name printed on them in a plastic envelope for storage. I felt so excited. I said thank you and told her it was a nice gift. She said, "Well, you are getting older." I couldn't understand why Aunt Joan said that, but Ma informed me I had insulted her. One more time I realized I did not have good social skills.

When I was about fifteen, I realized nothing I could ever do would make Ma happy. I picked her a big bouquet of lilacs from our bushes. She didn't go into the yard, and I thought she would like to have some in the house. She screamed at me that the smell bothered her, that it was suffocating her, and that she had emphysema.

When I was about seventeen, I realized for the second time that I could never make her happy. As Mother's Day was fast approaching, I went to Bing's Drugstore and saw four of the most beautiful cards I had ever seen. All had painted garden scenes, and each stood up like a panorama. I thought Ma would really like them, that maybe their beauty would make her happy, so I bought all four of them for her as a gift. At the same time, I bought something for myself, although I long ago forgot what it was. When Mother's Day arrived, I gave her the cards. She was furious; she spent most of her life being furious. I told her I thought she'd like them – I couldn't understand why she didn't. She asked me why I didn't buy her a gift, and I told her the beautiful cards were her gift. I explained that I didn't have money after buying her the cards, and what I needed to buy for myself, to buy her another gift. She started screaming at me, "You are always thinking of yourself. You spent money on yourself instead of buying a gift for me. You're selfish." Later that day, I heard her talking to one of her friends on the phone about the cards I had given her. She expressed outrage at my stupidity, and I felt embarrassed.

I never made her happy. And neither did Pa.

For years, Ma and Pa lived apart, and then, in his mid-50s, Pa developed congestive heart failure and was admitted to the hospital. He must have been in bad shape because when released, he was considered permanently disabled. He couldn't work or live alone anymore, so he came back to Ma's house, a thin, pathetic, filthy old drunk, and yet, only 55 years old. I remember wondering how the hospital staff had taken care of him without gagging. He stank of stale sweat and tooth rot. He had long fingernails, stained with nicotine. His jagged toenails had dirt under them. The hospital staff had put him in the whirlpool, and he loved it. I suspect they gave him that treat because no one wanted to physically clean him.

It was impossible to ignore Pa being back in the house. For one thing, Ma acted even less happy and more angry than her usual miserable self.

Pa had to stop drinking, so he dried out on the couch. During this process, he was a mess. He stank, his body shook and his face trembled, his eyes were wild, and his teeth were caked with white crud. He moaned and cried. He didn't shave for at least two weeks. At one point Ma said, "It will be over soon." I assumed she meant the withdrawal from a lifetime of alcohol abuse. Years later, I thought about her statement and wondered if she was waiting, hoping, for him to die on that couch.

One day, when Pa was starting to feel better, I had to go to the grocery store to do the shopping for Ma. I called out to Pa, "Do you want anything at the store?" As I walked into the room to hear this answer, I saw him lying on the couch, his sick bed, in a state of self-arousal.

It was a life-changing moment for me because I knew my only response to him was always obedience. He was the absolute and unquestioned authority in my life. Fortunately, he did not demand anything from me. But I realize how that day could have proceeded in a very different manner.

There existed one shred of sexual decency left in Pa, and I witnessed it that day. I was spared more horror at the hands of my parents.

What I was not spared, however, was an awareness that I would have done anything he wanted me to do. What a sad thing to realize that I would have submitted to a filthy skunk of a man because he had an iron will. That incident colored my relationships with all men who hold just authority over me.

Eventually, Pa dried out. It took months for the congestive heart failure to lessen, and he was never the man he had been before that disease. After his recovery, such as it was, he went from the couch to the little room behind the front hall which became his bedroom. For years after, he used his coat as a pillow, sleeping on the mattress with blankets and no sheets.

The weirdness in the house continued after Pa's "recovery." One day, Pa was standing near the open flame on the gas range in the house to get warm in the dead of winter. I came home from a date and Ma greeted me at the door saying, "Your father's back is gone." I wondered what she meant. It turns out, she was trying to tell me he had set his back on fire.

Pa would not go to the hospital by ambulance and had waited for me to come home to take him.

Before I could take him to the hospital this time, I had to listen to what had happened. Ma said his clothes had caught on fire, and she heard him scream, "Oh no!" He ran into the living room and rolled over onto the couch Ma slept on to smother the flames. She was furious that he had burned her bathrobe. She said he should have gotten on the floor to roll, and he said if he had done that, he wouldn't have been able to get the fire out. I agreed with him, and that made her furious with me, too.

The problem now was I had just parked my used red Chrysler in the driveway. The narrow, uphill driveway required a 90 degree turn to get into it, plus it had a chain-link fence that opened into it, making the space even more narrow. The Chrysler was my first car so backing it up was not one of my stronger skills, and to be honest, it still isn't. Usually, Pa would back it out in the morning so I could go to work, and I would park it on the street after work, and he would drive it into the driveway. I had just mastered pulling it into the driveway, but I had never backed it out onto the street.

I went out to the car and though it took some time, I managed to successfully back it out onto the street. I took Pa to the closest hospital, St. Joseph's. I felt morally superior to both Ma and Pa in that moment because I did not tell Pa to go to the hospital by cab. I actually took him, which is more than could be said for his care of me.

The Emergency Room staff took him into the back room as soon as they learned he had suffered serious burns. I do not know the details of what the doctors and nurses do to a person with a burned back. Pa was back there in the room quite a while, and I waited.

When they were through treating him at the hospital, he came home. I got the job of changing the bandages and dressing his back. I had never seen a serious burn before, and it was mean looking. For a week or ten days I dutifully changed the bandages as carefully as I could. It was a disgusting, filthy job that his wife, my mother, should have been doing. He stank. He and water had not only never made friends, but they had also never even made each other's acquaintance.

Even now, thinking of those bandages, I get squeamish.

At one point during the healing process Pa said, "I haven't said anything to your mother, but I think my back is infected." I told him I didn't think it was, and I later learned that I was right. I honestly had no idea whether it was infected or not; and truthfully, I didn't care either way.

Select Photographs

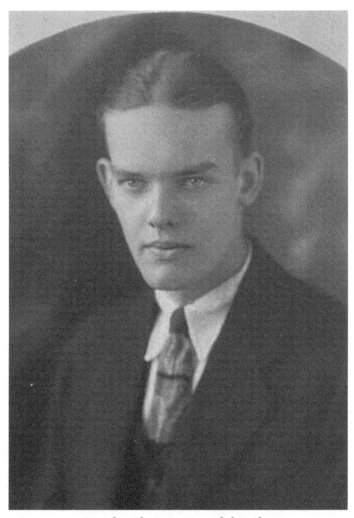

Pa when he was a model at the
Rhode Island School of Design

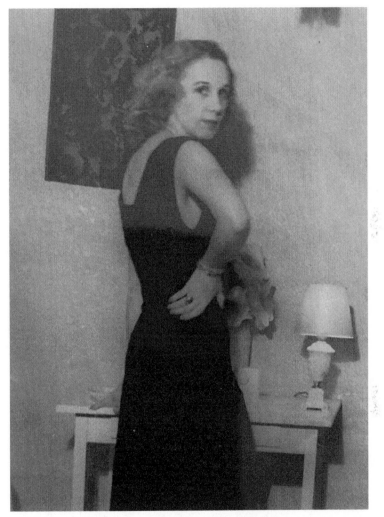

Ma when she was a model at the
Rhode Island School of Design

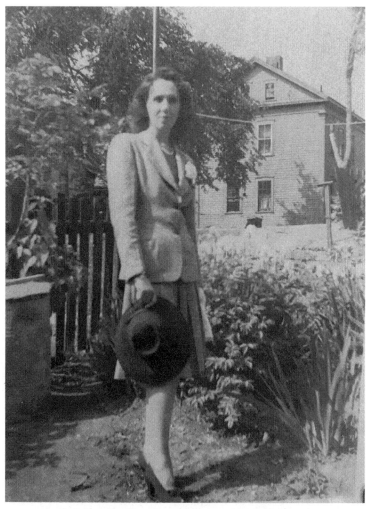

Ma in a family garden in Bristol, RI

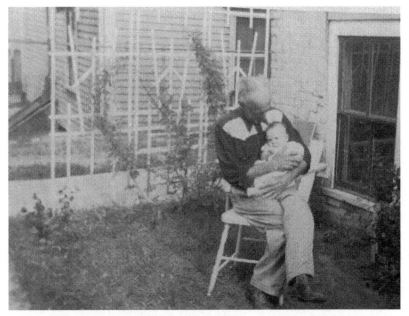

Grandpa Herb holding me and looking at me with love, about a
year after buying Ma chemicals to assist her in killing me.

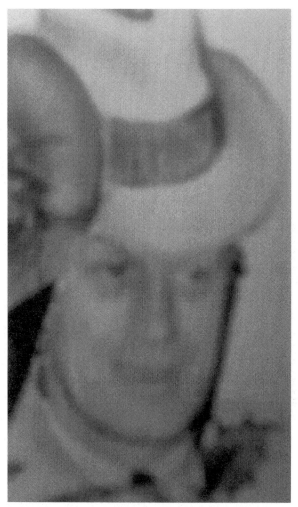

Uncle Sherman

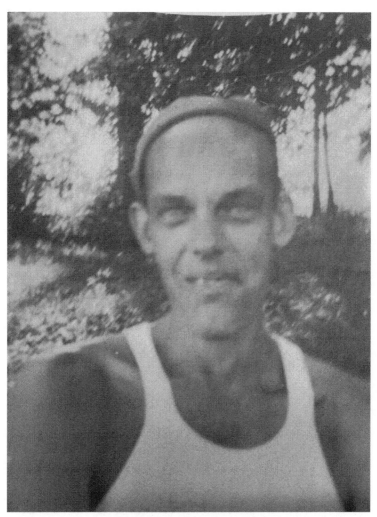

Pa on his land in Shun Pike.
Ma sold it behind his back for $500 in 1978.

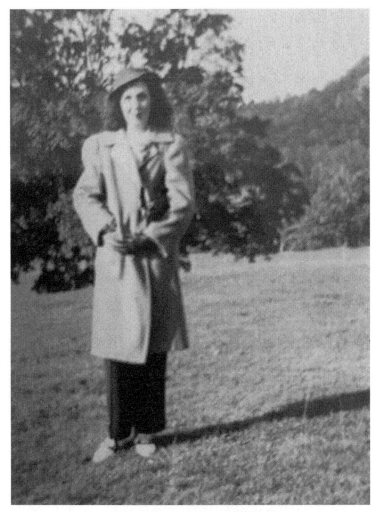

Ma approaching middle age.

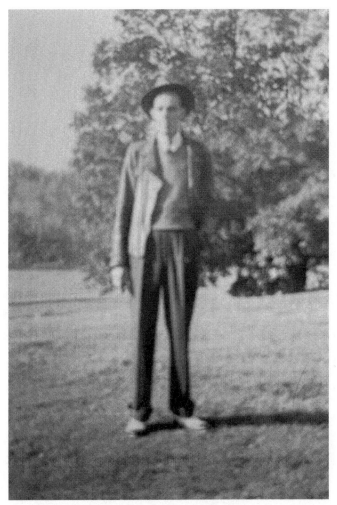

Pa approaching middle age.

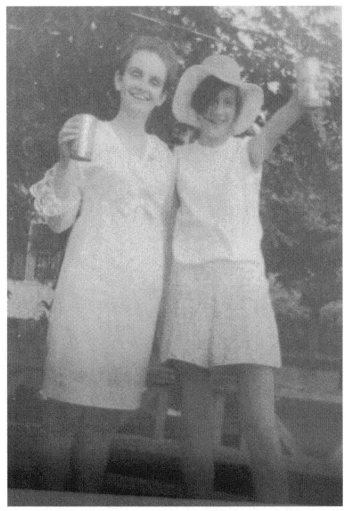

Cynthia (left) and Friend in Bristol, RI, for the Independence
Day Parade. Note Cynthia's facial structure.

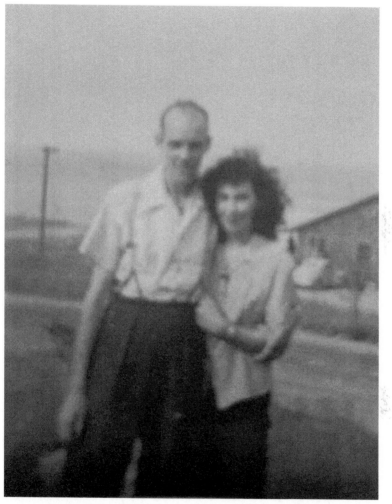

Pa and Ma when they were still on good terms.

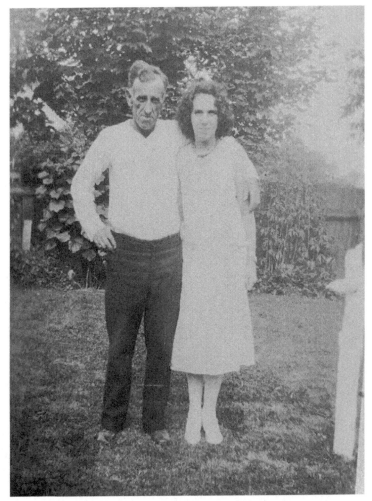

Grandpa Herb and Ma

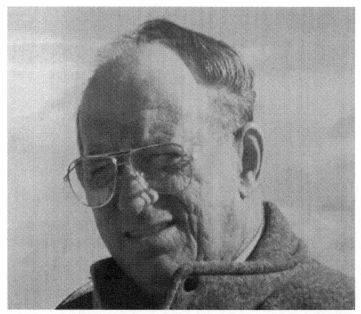

Jimmy Toolin (1935-2006). We were on an anniversary trip.

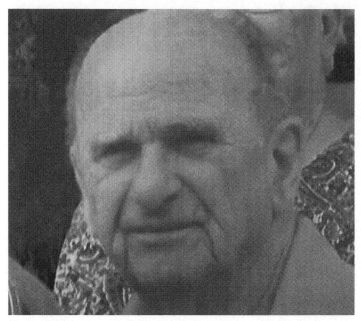

Bill Wilson (1935-) We were at a picnic with his friends.

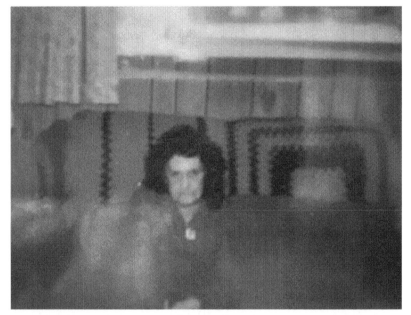

Ma at age 70.

Chapter 6

Science and Fiction

Pa and I had quite a few things in common. We both liked to make jams, jellies, and pickles; we liked the idea, although not the activity, of gardening; we liked antique cars; and for entertainment, we liked Western and Science Fiction books and shows. Pa introduced me to Zane Grey's Western novels, and I devoured all of them. As an adult, I took three trips out West and every time I saw a location that Zane Grey had mentioned, I was excited, as if I had been transported back in time to the Old West.

Before Pa left Ma and me, he and I used to watch an occasional science fiction show together, like *Twilight Zone*, *Outer Limits*, or *Lost in Space*. For years, whenever I had the opportunity, I used to say, "Danger, Will Robinson!" as if I were the Robot in that old television show. Liking science fiction led to an interest in space.

I was only seven when the Soviet Union successfully launched Sputnik, and Pa assumed that American power was on the decline. He seemed dejected. He explained the issues to me in language I understood. "The bad guys are the Russians, and they won the space race instead of us good guys, the Americans. That is really bad. We have to beat them in space next time." Pa and I were equally delighted with the advent of the United States' space program. When Alan Shepherd became the first man in space in 1961, and John Glenn orbited the globe on the Friendship 7 mission in 1962, and then Neil Armstrong, Michael Collins, and Buzz Aldrin went to the moon in 1969, we were ecstatic. We good guys beat the evil Russians.

I wish Pa and I had made the move from watching space events on the television, to going into the backyard more often to look at the night sky. Once he pointed out the Big Dipper to me, or at least what he thought was the Big Dipper, but I couldn't detect it. I imagined going into the desert – any desert in the world would have been fine – and lying on the hood of a car at night to see the stars in the sky. I knew I would see more there than I ever could in Providence, RI. Maybe I would have seen the Milky Way. I wondered if Pa ever saw it. I suspected he did because he was born before the city lights blurred the stars.

As an adult I fulfilled that wish. I looked at the sky in the Mojave Desert in the middle of the night. It was spectacular. I sat in a parked Mustang, with all the windows down, smelling the strange scents and listening to the silence of the desert. I looked up and saw more stars than I imagined existed. Yet I knew I was looking at a small area of the sky, on a little planet, on the outskirts of the Milky Way, a small spiral galaxy. I thought the universe is too large for a human to comprehend, but I was happy with the view of it I had that night.

Our common interest in space created a love of the universe in me that stays with me still. I wasn't just interested in our solar system, which at that time was thought to extend only to Pluto, but I wanted to know about galaxies, star and planet formation, asteroids, and interstellar travel. Pa gave me that love. I remember telling him one day that I wished I had been born later because I would not live long enough to know if there was life on other planets and if there were whether we would be able to communicate with alien life forms or not. As a child, I thought it would be so cool to be able to talk to someone from another planet and find out how they thought. It would be even better to date someone from another planet, assuming the aliens had gender.

Think of that! Intergalactic marriage! Maybe with someone who looked like Worf, the Klingon, or Spock, the Vulcan, both from *Star Trek*.

I remember the thoughts I had at that time and I am happy to have lived long enough to learn so many things about the solar system and outer space that we didn't know when I was young - that Pluto is on the inner boundary of the Kuiper Belt and that the outer boundary of the Oort Cloud is up to 1000 times more distant from the sun than are the planets.[2] And that planets exist in other solar systems, many light years away from

[2] Frank Summers, *New Frontiers: Modern Perspectives on Our Solar System*, Space Telescope Science Institute: The Great Courses.

this one.

After I married, not a Klingon warrior or a logical Vulcan, but a mere human, I decided to continue pursuing my bachelor's degree at the University of Massachusetts. The University required that students take some math and/or science courses to fulfill the general education requirement. I was nervous about taking these courses because I had not earned good grades in an earlier attempt at a college education. I noticed that there was a course called Astronomy for Non-Math Majors and I immediately registered for it. That professor opened the universe up for me. In one lecture, he showed us a slide of the night sky. I could see more stars than I could count and I wondered if any of them had planets around them like in our solar system, and, if so, about the possibility of intelligent life on them. Then he showed us a slide of the same area of the sky but magnified many times. He explained we had been looking at some stars, but most of the points of light visible on the unmagnified slide were galaxies. I thought that if this was a slide of one part of the sky, there must be many millions of galaxies, perhaps many billions. I wondered how many solar systems in each galaxy? How much intelligent life? There existed billions and billions and billions of stars, possibly trillions, in all of these galaxies. There had to be other life out there.

The professor then made the point that the slide we were looking at included just a small section of the sky. Even today, when I think of that lecture, I am amazed to think of the volume of the universe and the quantity and diversity of its contents.

One day I was looking at a popular magazine, probably *National Geographic*, while sitting in my primary care physician's waiting room. I flipped through the pages, making sure to avoid animal extinction and hunting pictures, and stopped at the space photos. As I turned the glossy pages, two things that I had never associated, came together in my mind. In my experience, the intersection of two or more unrelated things often sparks a new creative idea.

Looking at a picture of the Milky Way, and the amazing number of planets in the galaxy, I thought of Pa's affairs and I wondered if he had other children.

Once I began to think of Pa as having had other children than me, I couldn't stop thinking of it. Could I really be the only child? Why hadn't I asked this question before? Had Pa gotten women other than Ma pregnant? Had he made them get abortions? Or had he had other children? I felt sick as I considered the possibilities. My imagination spiraled out of control. Was that why he left us when I was 13? To be with another woman and his child? Or children? Had he had another family? I had always assumed he left because Ma was so mean and crazy. But now another possible explanation for his behavior faced me. I thought, *"Pa had another family, a happy one."* When he announced that he was moving, he was shaving at the bathroom sink, and he looked at me and said,

"One of the reasons I'm leaving is because I can't stand the faces you make." That is what I thought he said, what I remember him saying, but I wonder now if he really said, "One of the reasons I'm leaving is because I can't stand your face."

I had a hideous face, or to be more accurate, a hideous head. My head was too small for my body. My jaw and teeth were deformed. My left eye wandered so much I wondered why it didn't go around the back of my head and hit my right eye. One eyebrow was significantly higher than the other.

Maybe he had another child, one with an attractive face. I thought, "M*aybe he has a pretty daughter, not someone who looks like me. And maybe that daughter's mother didn't act crazy.*"

I thought about what I knew, and I came up with a set of assumptions. Pa married Ma at age 20, and Ma told me he cheated on her within one year of their getting married. She caught him. Ma was walking down the street, and Pa was so enthralled with a woman he was talking to that he didn't even see Ma approaching. I assume she heard what he was saying, and I imagine it to be the beginning of the end of Ma and Pa's marriage. Unfortunately, it took many long decades for the story of the sad relationship between them to play itself out.

A man who cheats on his new wife at age 21, and continued to do so with multiple women, multiple times, until he was too old and sick to attract women, must have made some of those women pregnant. And perhaps one or more of them, carried his child to full-term?

Ma had estimated that Pa had at least 200 girlfriends during their marriage. That number could be low, because they both told me, at different times, that after I was born in 1950 they never had relations again. Ma had already told me that he had cheated within a year of their marriage, and he told me he cheated after I was born. Ma also told me that one day after he became disabled, he sat at the kitchen table crying because "he couldn't get any more young girls."

Pa was a whoremaster. Both Ma and Pa confirmed this to me. Ma seemed appalled by it, and he was proud of it. No longer the handsome rakish rogue that he was when Ma fell in love with him, Pa was dirty, he stank, and he drank and smoked. How could a man who looked and smelled like him find a steady stream of women who would sleep with him? I can only conclude that as he deteriorated with age, he must have picked up prostitutes or desperate homeless women. Those extramarital affairs drove a wedge between him and Ma. They impacted me too – and eventually my family - because Ma never missed an opportunity to tell anyone who would listen that she had married a real dirtbag.

Something else about his behavior directly involves me. His secrecy infuriated me and continues to do so because he kept me in ignorance as to whether he ever had other children. I want to know if I have half-brothers or half-sisters. And if I do, are they still alive? I want to know if I have nieces or nephews, or grandnieces or grandnephews, that I don't know about. I wonder even now, *"Do I have any relatives at all?"*

I wish I had asked Pa before he died if he had other children, but I didn't. At the time it seemed to me that what he did in his life was his business. I felt I would be violating some code of secrecy or privacy if I asked him, "Were there other children?" I regret that I lacked the courage to ask him that question. I wonder even now, *"If I had asked, would he have told me the truth?"*

I regret not asking this question because I think it was my right to know the answer, and it was his duty to tell me the truth. I wonder how he would have answered. "Yes, I had five other children by as many women. Do you want their names and addresses?" Or "No, I always used birth control and I never made anyone besides your mother pregnant." At a deeper level, I regret my own insecurities. I wanted to know about other children, but I wanted to believe I was special, the only one, or the only one he cared enough about to give his name to: the only legitimate one.

And I regret not asking him the most important question of all, "Do you love me?"

I have spent numerous fruitless hours staring at a computer screen, using ancestry.com to look for a baby or babies born between 1928 and 1985, anywhere in New England, using combinations of Pa's first name, or one or both of his middle names, or initials, with his last name.

I think, *Almighty God in Heaven! Just one! By the love of all that is holy, let me find just one!* Nothing. No one. Nada. Zilch.

But what could I have expected? Would Pa really have acknowledged paternity on another child's birth certificate? I can imagine the fight he and Ma would have had if she ever saw such a legal document.

I know I must accept that if there are any relatives, I will probably never find them now.

I fantasize about what it would be like to find my relatives and meet them. Since Pa spent most of his life in Providence, I imagine Rhode Island people who have moved out of the city and into the suburbs. They probably own neat ranch houses, or white capes with black shutters, and a white picket fence around their yards. They have married children and grand-children, and everyone comes home for the Thanksgiving feast and the July 4 clambake. There could be whole clans of children born to my father since 1928 and it would be such fun to meet them and get to know them. We would share common interests, and I would be part of their families, and they of mine.

I dream sometimes about a hesitant knock on the door, an email or letter, or most probably, a phone call. I would answer, thinking it was one of my friends and instead hear… "Are you Cynthia? I don't know how to say this, but I think we might be related. I was on ancestry.com the other night and I got a leaf to your tree. I think your father might be my grandfather." And I would scream into the phone, "Yes! Yes! I always knew in my heart that you existed. I could feel that I was not alone on this planet." And we would start a relationship and enjoy each other's company. Just like a real family.

I think, then, of how long ago 1928 was – over 90 years ago. If Pa had a child in 1928, that child would probably be long dead by now. But maybe that child married and had children and grandchildren who would still be alive. Stranger things have happened! *Dream, Cynthia, dream. Don't give up the search.*

There has to be at least one half-sibling, or the child of that half-sibling, alive and well. Maybe there are many. I wonder, *will I ever know?*

Chapter 7

Life with Ma and Pa on Till Street

When I married Jimmy, we had a small reception at a friend's house. The perfect venue.

It was an old farmhouse, with access to the gardens. Friends could take food from the buffet table and sit on antique furniture or wander through the gardens. Though younger than I am now, Pa came to the reception. He remained a filthy old man in the baggy clothes he wore every day. At least he tried to make himself presentable by shaving. Pa stayed long enough to hear the toast. Ma didn't attend at all. I felt surprised that Pa attended, even for a short time, but I was not surprised that Ma stayed at home. When I graduated from high school, Ma and Pa came to the ceremony, but left early.

My Jimmy did not take offense at Pa's short visit or Ma's absence. They would not have fit in. Jimmy knew people would ask me what was wrong with them. He recognized that they were people comfortable living in the underclass, and he knew the dire straits of their circumstances.

Jimmy wanted to help Ma and Pa. He was the kind of man

who rescued stray people, gave bums his last dollar, and bought sandwiches for the homeless. We discussed them coming to live with us in Connecticut. I argued strongly not to invite them to live with us. I knew that if they moved in with us, they would remain in the underclass and slowly pull our middle-class lifestyle down to their level.

We owned a nice 1200 square foot ranch house on a postage stamp sized lot. Looking at the house from the sidewalk, I would say it looked neat. The front lawn, though small, had a red maple in the middle of it, and an asphalt driveway. A chain link fence enclosed the back yard, which held a tiny shed, and three apple trees, a lilac bush, and two maple trees. Our dog, Columbo, patrolled the border from morning to night.

I thought I finally had a happy home.

I knew if Ma and Pa moved in, our happy home would become a war zone. Jimmy expressed concern for Ma and Pa's safety. He pointed to the fact we had enough bedrooms for everyone and a full cellar where they could store a few special possessions. Jimmy insisted that we bring them from Burnham Street to Till Street. Eventually, he wore me down. I gave in to Jimmy's wishes within the first year of our marriage, and the process of the move began.

Pa sold the house on Burnham Street to one of his neighbors, Ricky, who lived in a third-floor walkup apartment two houses away. Pa started packing things up in boxes. On moving day, Ricky brought their furniture, their three cats and a dog, and approximately 70 boxes of "special possessions." The boxes went into the cellar along with the majority of their furniture. I looked at Jimmy; he looked uncomfortable, like a man beginning to realize he might have made a mistake. I refused to take any of the blame for the beginning of our melded household, so I smiled at Jimmy and said, "You did this to us."

The first day that Ma and Pa arrived, the battle lines were drawn. Ma refused to sleep in the same room as Pa. Ma slept in the room next to us, and Pa slept in the added bedroom on the other side of the house. Ma kept her cat, Whitey, in her room; Pa kept his cats, Singapore and Bangladesh, in his room. Pierre, the poodle, stayed in the dining room.

Pa put down two litter boxes in his bedroom, and one in Ma's bedroom. He thought buying cat litter was a waste of money, so he used ripped up newspaper in the boxes instead. Then he put newspaper on the hardwood dining room floor so Pierre could urinate and move his bowels. Each animal had a collar with about a five-foot piece of clothesline that attached it to a piece of furniture.

Then Pa brought a metal bedpan to Ma for her to use in her bedroom, even though she was not ten feet from the only bathroom. And Pa put an empty gallon milk jug in his bedroom, with the cover, to use as a urinal. Just like on Burnham Street, he used his coat for a pillow, and used blankets but no sheets. Pillows and sheets were available; he just didn't want them.

What had once been a comfortable home with sufficient space began to feel crowded to Jimmy. It felt claustrophobic to me.

Jimmy worked as a bus driver. Within a few weeks I noticed that he had started spending more time working. I understood his absence because I felt the need to be out of the house, too. I was studying for my BA in sociology; I started spending a lot of time at school and at my part-time job as a retail security guard.

Ma was jealous of the relationship I had with Jimmy, and I think, of me. Ma had never learned how to cook well, although she had attempted to make a good meal once in a while. The only memorable meals came at Thanksgiving. I had had cookies and milk for breakfast every morning until I moved out on my own. I remember dinners of spaghetti sauce over potatoes and Chef Boyardee canned ravioli or spaghetti.

After I married Jimmy, Ma would bake Jiffy cakes for him. I think she hoped he would like her. I think she tried to impress him. Not to be outdone by Ma, I enrolled in a Wilton cake decorating class to learn how to decorate cakes like a professional. It gave me a great deal of pleasure to show her my cakes – they were better than hers, made from scratch and not out of a box that cost 10 cents.

Ma spent her time knitting. She made zigzag afghans, one of which I still have, and fake mink hats. She made the mink hats with black and white angora yarn. I began to wonder if minks came in black and white stripes. It alarmed me that anyone could look at a knit hat made from angora yarn, and think the hat was knit from a dead mink? A live mink, if it came across one of those hats, would not run away in fear of losing its life. She also loved to make pink poodle covers for rolls of toilet tissue and nail polish bottles. I thought, *pink is a color no self-respecting poodle would ever be,* but Ma apparently did not realize this. In response to her knitting, I became a master crocheter. I don't know why I was competitive with Ma because she was inadequate in everything she tried to do, especially cooking and knitting. Yet I felt this desire to show her that I could easily do everything she did, and I would produce a better product.

Ma always said I had no social skills, although she didn't use that phrase as it would be too advanced for her level of schooling. I think she said – "You don't know anything!" – in her shrill, derisive voice. At that time, she was right. I didn't have any social skills, but that was because she never taught them to me. In hindsight, Ma could not pass on what she didn't have herself.

Ma had gone to grammar school with her friend Christy, and they had stayed in touch by phone over the decades, and on occasion Christy would come to the Burnham Street house.

Christy came to lunch at my Till Street house when Ma and Pa were living with us. I don't remember what I served for lunch, but I had made a cake for dessert. Christy brought a tomato soup cake. I thought it was a gift and served the cake I had made. Ma started screaming at me in front of Christy, "Don't you know anything? You are so ignorant. Aren't you going to serve her cake?"

Now I know that I should have served her cake. But then, I did not. However, I did know it was impolite to scream at me in front of Christy. During that incident, I thought I could teach Ma more about manners than she ever taught me.

This incident was somewhat like the time in Providence when a neighbor took us to a restaurant. I was about ten or twelve years old. It was probably my first time in a restaurant. When the salad came, I smelled it. God only knows why I did that; I certainly don't. Ma turned to me and said, "If you are going to act like that, you'll never go to another restaurant." I didn't know it was impolite to smell food when it was served in a restaurant. But I thought, *"Ma, you are being rude again."*

Ma didn't take showers or baths and continued to wash in the bathroom sink even though our Till Street bathroom had a tub and shower with running hot and cold water. The bathroom was set up like those of many ranch houses – first a vanity sink, then a toilet, and last, a tub/shower combo with a shower curtain. It was as if she had moved the bathroom from Burnham Street to the house on Till Street. The difference was that our bathtub faucets had hot and cold water attached to them.

Once or twice a year Ma would stand at the bathroom sink

and I would wash her hair in it, not three feet from the shower and tub. Then every three or four months she would stand at the sink and I would wash her back. But she would never consider getting into the tub. I started to fantasize about her being the Wicked Witch of the West, the one that melted when Dorothy threw water on her to put out a fire. At least in our Till Street bathroom, we didn't have to heat water on the kitchen stove, and we could rinse her hair easily.

At one point Ma decided she wanted me to cut her hair. I told her I didn't know how to cut hair - I wasn't a hairdresser. She said, "It's easy, just cut it." So, I did. I could feel the grease in my hands as I cut strand after strand of long white and grey hair off her head. Of course, it looked horrid and I heard her say to Pa, "She ruined my hair." And he answered, "Yes, she did." I wondered, did anyone really look at her hair before?

By this time, Ma had taken to wearing black polyester wigs with hair that cascaded down to her shoulders. One had to lift up the plastic hair to get to her filthy, smelly, greasy hair.

Pa also maintained the same kind of hygiene as he had at the Burnham Street house, although I never had to wash him. He would use the same face cloth and towel for months. Every few days, when I did the laundry, I would ask him for them, but he always refused to let me wash them. The face cloth would be so stiff with dirt it looked like a terry cloth sculpture. Pa never, to my knowledge, brushed his teeth, which were coated with a mealy substance before they started falling out.

At least he shaved somewhat regularly.

One day Jimmy told me he had overheard a conversation between Ma and Pa. Pa wondered how the shower worked, and Ma told him, "It can't be that hard to figure out. Ask Jimmy." Pa never did ask but hearing about that conversation told me what I had already suspected: neither Ma nor Pa had ever taken a shower or a bath in a tub. Never, not even once in their lives.

But what I had to deal with every night in the kitchen was much worse than the personal hygiene, or lack thereof, in the bathroom. I would make dinner for the family, and Pa would make dinner for himself and then something for Ma. It wasn't that I wouldn't cook for them, rather Ma would only eat what Pa cooked. And Pa never wanted to eat what I cooked. Pa would make Minute Rice, and beef or chicken, for himself, and plain hot water to drink, which he insisted was "every bit as good as tea." He cooked his meat in the toaster oven. Ma would usually eat one hot dog cooked in the oven at 350 degrees for half an hour, and maybe a piece of bread. Every night as I set the table, Pa, who was by then in a wheelchair, would roll over to Ma's bedroom and say, "Are you ready to eat?" and she always said, "No, not yet." So, he would cook his own meal at the same time as I would prepare ours. As soon as we all sat down to eat, Ma would call out and say, "I think I'm ready to eat now." Pa would leave his food at the table, swearing like a trooper, and make her meal. This little scenario played out every night for years.

It is lucky that Ma did this with Pa and not me. I would have gone in and said to her, "I am preparing my meal now, and when it is done, I am going to eat. If you want to eat before I have completed my meal, you should have me cook it now. If you don't, you will have to wait until I am finished." But Pa never said anything like that. I used to fantasize about going out to eat – to dinner, to a restaurant, to a friend's house – during their nightly encounter.

One day Pa decided he didn't want chicken or beef in the toaster oven, so he made beef stew for himself. He was telling me about it, and I stood listening. Ma hobbled out to the kitchen and said, "She doesn't care about that!" So, Pa went to the kitchen sink and poured the entire pot of beef stew down the garbage disposal.

He was a skinny old man, angry, and I suppose, hurt by what Ma said and by what he incorrectly thought I was thinking. Ma could never have enough revenge for his adultery: relentless, unforgiving, eternal revenge. I would think, "Shut up, Ma. Give us a break! You are ruining everyone's life!"

There were worse things that went on at that kitchen sink than beef stew going down the garbage disposal.

Pa's bedroom was on one side of the house, beyond the kitchen and dining room, and the one bathroom was on the opposite side. I guess he decided it was too far to go from his bedroom to the bathroom to relieve himself. He kept a gallon milk jug under his bed to urinate in, and he capped it and stored it until it was full. Then he would empty it. I fervently hoped he emptied the jug in the toilet and not in the kitchen sink. But I'm afraid that if the bathroom was too far to roll in the middle of the night, it would have been too far to roll if he was carrying a gallon of urine.

Pa tried to help me maintain the house so he would do the dishes. One day I came into the house from the screened porch where he put his dry underwear to "air them out" and his nose was running from his nostrils into the dishwater. He continued to wash the dishes in the same water.

I think of that kitchen sink, its drain not clogged with bits of food and grease but coated with urine and snot.

Ma and Pa stopped drinking while they still lived on Burnham Street, but I believe my mother frequently longed for a drink. Years after she quit, when I was a young wife, I made a rum cake dessert. I poured too much rum into the measuring cup. I became distracted, talking to Ma since she was in the kitchen instead of in her self-exiled bedroom. As I poured the extra rum back into the bottle she said, "If it was me, I would have drunk the extra." She would have drunk it all, probably licking the measuring cup dry and then proceeding on to any rum left in the bottle.

It made me sad to think back on how Ma and Pa drank. Ma was a mean drunk and so was Pa, but her father, my Grand-father Herb, was a happy drunk. If it wasn't for him, I would have assumed all drunks are mean. By the time they lived with us on Till Street, Ma and Pa were dry alcoholics, behaving just as they had as mean drunks on Burnham Street. That meanness made them fight.

When they moved in with us Ma decided she wanted to be financially independent. To achieve this, Ma and Pa agree to split his social security check after common living expenses had been paid. I assumed he knew this would never work.

From her half of the remainder, Ma had to pay for her own medications and other minor expenses. By the end of the month, she was broke. She couldn't even afford her medications, and she seemed discouraged. I remember her saying she couldn't make it on her own. I imagine her finding out that she remained financially dependent on Pa didn't help them get along. It just gave them more to fight about.

Pa also seemed discouraged about money. Once Pa told me that Ma had spent every cent he had. I thought, although I never dared to say, *"After you paid for your other women?"* I suspect Ma did it on purpose. She made him pay, literally, for his adulterous behavior.

The only times Ma didn't want to fight were during thunderstorms. After moving to Connecticut, she would watch the news for the weather. She came to call our area Thunderstorm Alley. When it stormed, at the first sign of thunder, Ma would hobble to Pa's room as fast as she could, as if he could protect her. It seemed like the height of hypocrisy.

At all other times, she couldn't get far enough away from him.

Ma wore a lot of jewelry. She had silver bangle bracelets that Pa had made for her when he was a metal worker and a gold plater, and a silver watch ring he had bought. When they had their 50th wedding anniversary, Pa bought her a diamond ring. He had given her one for their engagement and now he gave her another. Every week he would go downtown – someone would give him a ride – and he would put more money on the ring. Ma did not know why he was leaving the house. So, every week when he left she would scream at him, "You took a young girl away from her home," the implication being he was going out to see an old whore. I don't know why he bought the ring. To surprise her? To please her? To make up for what he had done to her? As far as I know, Ma never apologized for the verbal abuse and by then she had crippling arthritis in her hands. She couldn't wear the ring.

I came home from work on their 50th Wedding Anniversary and did one of the worst things I ever did. I am not proud of it and it was one of the most telling moments of my relationship with Ma. She said, "Couldn't you have at least bought me a single red rose for my anniversary?" She said it quiet and gentle, like she was confused by the lack of a present. I imagine she had been expecting something, maybe a nice gift. I gave her the gift of brutal honesty as she had once given it to me about the abortion attempt. I didn't plan what to say. It just came out: I said, "What are you talking about? All I've ever heard from you is that you hate him and wish you hadn't married him. If I was going to buy you anything it would have been a sympathy card." She looked at me like she finally understood – eyes big and sad. She let the air out of her lungs. She pursed her lips together and said, "Ohhhh," long and quiet. I turned and walked away.

What I said was cruel. I think the anger had been building in me for decades. I wish I hadn't said that to her, but I also hadn't planned it. To me, she was unbelievable. Why celebrate something that you never said a good word about with someone you said nothing but bad things about?

I wondered if that is what happened with me. Did Ma not mean to tell me about her attempt to kill me? Perhaps it just slipped out?

I wonder if she told Pa what I said that day, when they talked late at night. Jimmy and my bedroom was at the end of the hall next to the bathroom. Ma's room was next. She said she was too weak to make it to the bathroom. She would urinate and defecate in a metal bedpan all day and cover it with one single sheet of paper towel. After Jimmy and I went to bed, Pa would roll over to her room and sit outside her open door with the bedpan, full of day-old stool floating in urine, on his lap. He sat there as if he could smell nothing, or as if her body waste smelled like fresh roses. They would talk, sometimes for a half hour or more, and then he would roll down the hall to the bathroom and empty the bedpan. He never cleaned it before he returned it to her. This nightly ritual drove Jimmy crazy, but because of my upbringing in Burnham Street, I thought nothing of it.

Ma did not age well. She stooped, doubled over because she had broken a disk in her back. She suffered from rheumatoid arthritis and osteoporosis. As a young woman, she had refused to drink or eat anything with calcium in it because, she said, milk made her sick. While that may have been true, I believe all her skeletal issues worsened because she did not eat much, and she drank so much. Half deaf and almost blind, Ma had a hunch back and a big belly. Her always-swollen feet looked like pig's feet. But her worst health problems were emphysema and heart disease.

I often thought back to when Ma and Pa lived on Burnham Street, both hospitalized for different ailments, about a day apart, in the same hospital. They had separate rooms on the same floor. When visiting, I would go visit one in one room, and then walk down the hall and see the other in another room. A nurse noticed and asked me what I was doing. When I explained that both of my parents were there, she became very upset about them being separated. The nurse thought she would please them by putting them in the same room. Ma set her straight, practically spitting out the words – "I won't be in the same room with that man!" The nurse just looked at my mother and then to me. I did the only thing I could think of; I shrugged and looked down at the floor.

The emphysema got worse when Ma lived on Till Street. Going to the doctor's office was an experience because Ma insisted on going in a special side door so she wouldn't have to walk past the people in the waiting room. The doctor's staff always gave her special treatment. They seemed to think her a sweet old lady, maybe a little eccentric because she wore a black polyester wig. I always hoped one of them would not go out of the way to please her so they would find out she was not a nice little old lady, but a rather miserable bitch. It never happened.

We went to the doctor once when she had a cold. The doctor gave her some medicine and I took her home. Once there, I gave her a pill and she looked at me, terrified, and said, "Are you trying to kill me?" I thought she was kidding, but she wasn't. Jimmy saw this exchange and said she wasn't acting right and that he thought she belonged in the hospital. I took her back to the doctor who thought she was fine. I told him about her comment, and I insisted she wasn't right. I argued with him on her behalf until he finally admitted her to the hospital. I thought, *"How odd is this? I am fighting for the life of a woman who tried to kill me..."*

Ma was admitted to the hospital and put on oxygen, which she would be on for the rest of her life. Jimmy got a long oxygen cord so she would be able to come out of her room though she never did when we were home. Jimmy told me that sometimes he would come home unexpectedly, and she would be sitting on the couch in the living room. As soon as he came in the front door, she would scurry into her bedroom. Scurry was the specific word he used, and it was a precise definition of her movement. Jimmy said that he pleaded with her to stay in the living room, but she refused. I used to try to get her to come out of her bedroom too or I'd go into her room to try to talk to her, both of which were impossible. Ma would never come out, and any attempt at conversation always ended with her yelling, telling me I was stupid and worthless, or complaining that I wasn't a good daughter.

One day I came home and found Jimmy very angry. The visiting nurse, who had been coming to the house since Ma came out of the hospital, had waited to see Jimmy. The nurse told him she wanted to know why we made Ma stay in her room. I don't know if Ma lied because she was malicious or told the story because she thought it was true; if her mind was finally starting to fail her, or if she wanted attention and sympathy. Regardless of the reason, she told a lie that could have gotten Jimmy and me in heaps of trouble with the government agencies who were caring for her.

While she lived with us, Ma always complained, saying things like, "I hoped I wouldn't wake up this morning." Or, "I hoped I would wake up dead." In my stupidity, I thought I would be able to make her feel better by pointing out that the way she felt had less to do with any particular disease, and more to do with the natural aging process. So, I said, "Ma, the aches and pains you have are probably because you are getting old." She became furious that I said that. She said, "That's a nice thing to say to your mother!" I thought, "*Ma! Do you even know what that word 'mother' means?"* In her mind, she wasn't old. She remained that beautiful woman, a model. Or at least someone who could regain that beauty if she worked at it. And I think she thought she had been a wonderful mother.

On the rare occasions when she talked, she always had Bristol on her mind. Born there in the early 1900s, Ma was not born well-to-do, yet I think her family had a more genteel life than my father's family, hailing from the Germany-France border to Boston by way of Nova Scotia and Maine. A small town on the bay, Bristol's sole claim to fame was the July 4th celebration. I think Ma liked that town because people there cared about her when she was young. Maybe that was always the issue: Ma wanted to be with people who cared about her.

Chapter 8

Senior Living and Death

Jimmy couldn't take Ma and Pa living in the house anymore. What I told him after we got married came true; they were destroying the house, ruining our lives, crucifying our peace. One night he told me that I had a choice to make. I could decide to have Ma and Pa continue to live on Till Street and Jimmy would leave us; or I could have Jimmy stay and Ma and Pa would have to leave. I was sickened by this choice.

The only reason Ma and Pa lived in our house was that he had insisted that they do so. I had warned him of the consequences, but he had stubbornly refused to listen to me. He kept saying they were old people, living in a run-down, dangerous neighborhood, under terrible conditions. He had been right. They didn't have heat or hot water, they didn't have bathing facilities, and yes, Pa had to sit on the front porch every July 4th to protect the house. Every Fourth at least one car would be burned up in the middle of the street.

But I knew things he didn't know, and no matter how hard I tried to tell him or how many times I explained the situation, he would not listen.

They were white trash. They would destroy the house on Till Street just like the one they destroyed on Burnham Street. They would bring everything they owned with them, including the animals. They would continue to fight with each other on a daily, sometimes even an hourly, basis. But most importantly, they would miss Providence. Providence was their home. They would miss their doctors, their pharmacy, their grocery store, and their neighborhood. They would miss having their own house. And they would miss their independence.

Now Jimmy had changed his mind, deciding he couldn't take it anymore, even though it was clear neither one of them was going to live much longer. It struck me as odd that now he knew I was right. Everything I had warned him about had come true. Even though I had no use for Ma and Pa, I felt no joy at being proven correct. I did not think it was right to make them face a move to a new location so late in their lives.

I had made the same mistake my mother had made. Because I was working on an advanced degree, I was financially dependent on Jimmy, at least until I could finish my graduate work. So, I had to choose not only between marriage and divorce, Ma and Pa staying or leaving, but also between finishing graduate school and being able to earn a living, or not being able to finish my degree and living in poverty.

It was a bad mistake Jimmy made the day he gave me that choice, as bad as the day he succeeded in convincing me to let him bring Ma and Pa to Connecticut. I remained married to Jimmy until the day he died. I took care of him through terminal cancer, and I held him as he died. I continued to love him, but I never cared for him with the same intensity as I had before he gave me those options. We fought more and loved less. I lost a lot of respect for him that day because of the choices he put in front of me. I was aware that he knew I had no choice any more than Ma had a choice to stay with her adulterous husband. She needed him to support her, just as I needed Jimmy to support me. That respect never came back.

I looked at Ma and Pa's age and condition, and my age and condition. They were both in their 70s and decrepit. They looked much older than they were. Pa had congestive heart failure and arthritis so bad his fingers bent to the side like clipped wings on a bird. He was in a wheelchair. Ma was partially bedridden, had a bad heart and emphysema, osteoporosis and arthritis, and was almost blind and half deaf. She was constantly on oxygen. I used to think that with the amount of drinking they both did, their guts should be pickled. They should have lived forever. I was young and healthy, with a family and a mortgage and a school loan. I chose for myself.

Maybe if there had been a relationship between us, I would have chosen Ma and Pa over Jimmy, but there wasn't and I didn't. They would have to find other housing and leave Till Street, and I would remain married and finish graduate school. I told Jimmy he should stay, but he would have to be the one to tell Pa. His eyes brightened up when I told him that; I could tell he thought I had chosen him over Ma and Pa, and that I loved him more than them. But he was wrong. What I really thought was, *"Silly man, I don't love my parents. I only do for them what I do because of duty. And now I don't love you as much as I did a day ago."*

Jimmy said he would tell Pa the next day, and that he would give them all the time they needed to find a place to live. I decided I would be absent from the house when this occurred, so I stayed at school as long as I could. When I came home, it was almost dark. The house was still and quiet, and the emotional temperature was colder than it had ever been. I walked from the front door into the bedroom and stayed there. Jimmy told me that Pa had said he and Ma would be out by the end of the following week, and they were. They moved into a small senior apartment about five miles from the house.

I know they were hurt. Pa was mad and Ma was insulted. She always thought she was better than Jimmy and his family, whom she referred to as lace curtain Irish. I never knew what she meant by that phrase, but I knew it wasn't good. She had always thought of her first home, the town of Bristol, RI, as being the epitome of fine living.

I never knew what the turning point was for Jimmy. Was it the constant bickering between Ma and Pa? The fact that Ma and Pa were filthy? That the cats and dog were filthy? That the house was always messy? That Pa would sit in his wheelchair outside of our room and talk to Ma, even when intimate moments were occurring in our bedroom? I asked Jimmy once what had been the culminating factor, but I know he didn't tell me the truth when he answered. He said he needed one of their bedrooms, so he had to ask them to go. I thought, *"Lying sack of shit. Be honest with them. Be honest with me."*

I don't know why I was surprised that Jimmy had finally had enough of Ma and Pa. No normal person could live in the conditions in that house forever. But that was the point. It wasn't going to be forever. They were almost dead.

And I don't know why Ma and Pa were surprised either. Did they think anyone else in the world lived like them? Had they sunk so low they didn't realize they were not normal?

No one won that day.

The day they moved out I got up early and went to school. I didn't say goodbye to anyone. I just got in my car and drove to U Mass and spent the day working on my dissertation. I returned well after dark. Both of their rooms were filthy. Pa had left his hernia belt and an empty gallon jug that he used to urinate in on this bedroom floor. Ma's room had balled up toilet tissue on the floor. They had left their cats. They had left all their boxes in the cellar but had taken the furniture they had been using in their rooms. I do not know how they got it moved. I never asked.

Ma and Pa had done the same thing on Till Street as on Burnham Street. They put collars on their animals and tied them on a short piece of clothesline rope. When I asked Pa why they did this, he said because they loved the animals and didn't want them to get outside and get hurt or killed.

Because they were on ropes, they went to the bathroom inside the house.

Pierre, the poodle that Ma thought had belonged to either one of Pa's girlfriends or a girlfriend's child, was tied in the dining room between the kitchen and Pa's bedroom. Pierre had a single layer of newspaper on the hardwood floor to use as his toilet. Although he was a little dog, he urinated a lot. We finally convinced Pa that the dog had to go. We put him to sleep. There was no way that dog would ever have been normal after living on a rope for years. The hardwood floor was permanently stained.

One of Ma's cats stayed in her room, also on a rope. Whitey had to be put to sleep because he developed cancer. We buried him in the backyard, at Ma's request, in his litter box. That seemed an odd thing to use as a casket for an animal you loved.

When they moved out, they left other cats behind. Those cats had slept with Pa where they had been on ropes in Pa's room for a few years. Like Pierre, the cats would never be normal animals. I took them off their ropes and pushed them so they would walk beyond a few feet. They returned to the ends of their ropes and sat on or near them. Finally, I took the cats to the veterinarian and had them put to sleep. One day Pa called and asked Jimmy how the cats were.

He said, "They're all dead." I thought, *Jimmy, you are a*

horse's ass. There was a better way of telling Pa that."

Pa called me and told me I had executed his cats. For weeks there was no communication between Ma and Pa and me. It was a time of great peace for me. I hated it when they started talking to me again. Jimmy called Pa and asked him if I could go visit my mother. He said he thought I should see her because I hadn't talked to her in weeks. Pa happily said yes. I thought, *"Mind your own business, Jimmy! Let me live in peace."*

After the cats were gone, we went in to assess how much damage Pa had done. We turned the thermostat up – Pa's room and the dining room had a separate heating system because they were an addition – and the bedroom filled with the greasy smell of burning cat urine.

Apparently, the cats didn't always make it to the litter box because sometimes a rope would get tangled around a furniture leg.

We had a carpenter come in to replace the floor, both the hardwood and the plywood subflooring. As he started to tear up the floor, he came out and told us he had some bad news. The cat urine had not only ruined the floor, but it had also wicked up the insulation in the walls. He had to remove all the drywall and insulation, and the electric heater. He said we were lucky that the urine had not wicked all the way up to the ceiling.

The more work he did, the worse the smell became. Finally, everything was out of the room, and he started reconstructing it. He put in new insulation, new drywall, new subflooring, and a new floor. Jimmy bought a new electric heater and had it put in. I cannot imagine the stories that carpenter must have told the other carpenters when they met for morning coffee.

In hindsight, I do not understand why I did not know this was happening. The only time I had gone in Pa's room was to clean it when he was in the hospital. I knew it was filthy. When I found a plastic milk jug half filled with his urine under his bed, I knew things weren't going well. Once I had called a carpenter to come to the house and give an estimate for the addition of a bay window in the living room. When the carpenter arrived, Pa rolled out of his room and it was as if an invisible trail of cat stink followed him. I could see that the carpenter was disgusted, and I was appalled. But I never realized how bad things had gotten until they moved out.

I should have gone to see them the day they moved out of Till Street, to make sure they were all right, but I just couldn't do it. It was as if every last ounce of life had been drained out of me, every last breath. I could not drive the few miles to their new residence.

The senior complex was composed of several single floor buildings, with multiple units in each, arranged in a row. Ma and Pa had a unit with a kitchen/living room combination, one bedroom large enough for two beds, and a bathroom.

A year later, Ma died. She always wore open toe slippers, and as she walked through the unit, she caught the toe of the slipper under the edge of their braided rug. She tripped and fell, breaking her hip. Her heart was so bad that the hospital did nothing with her hip, and only tried to stabilize her. They could not operate.

Jimmy took me to see her, and she was in rough shape. She knew us but was otherwise incoherent. She was in a semiprivate room. Her roommate was in her bed, praying the Rosary even though she had no beads. My mother looked at me with fear in her eyes and said, "Wait until your father gets home. He is going to be mad when he sees this strange woman in our living room." I told her it was okay, that he wouldn't be upset. She kept raving about it. When it was time to go, I believe I kissed her on the cheek, probably the first time I had ever done it. I don't know if I said, "I love you," which I would have said because it is something you are supposed to say to a dying parent. I might have just said, "I will see you tomorrow," or, "Goodbye."

We left and the next day Pa called me at work and said, "The worst has happened. Your mother has died. When the nurse went in this morning, she was gone." I said okay, and I would be at his place soon.

Pa arranged Ma's funeral. She was buried in Bristol, which I think would have made her happy. She loved Bristol. She never should have left it.

After her funeral, I cleaned out her closet. I went through her pockets because I didn't want to accidentally throw out anything that might mean something to me later. She had two one-dollar bills to her name, in a cheap polyester jacket that reeked of Avon Persian Woods cologne. I kept her jewelry and the two dollars and put them in a drawer. I assume I still have them, somewhere.

I often wondered what happened to her. I think Ma was born to be an ornament – she was the beloved daughter of a working-class couple in a sea town. I have a picture of her when she was a baby, old enough to just start sitting up. She had the most beautiful smile on her face. Ma had been a happy little girl. Somewhere along the line she stopped being happy. She expected to be her husband's cherished ornament. How sad. I wonder, did she lose her mind because of Pa's adultery? Or had his cheating made her a miserable person, full of hatred and the desire for revenge. I suspect the latter. She verbally abused Pa and me for decades. I can understand how she felt about Pa, but not about me. All I did was live, and she had only her own fear of death to blame for that.

Pa died six weeks after Ma in October of the same year. In the time between their deaths a lot happened. Pa wanted to visit Ma's grave on their wedding anniversary, a three-hour drive away. He wanted to go to Nova Scotia, where some of his family had lived decades before. His father emigrated from there before Pa was born, and Pa had visited there as a boy. He even planned the route. And he wanted to go back to Florida, where he told me he had "ridden the rails and been a hobo." He said he was proud he had ridden the rails, like it was a free and independent lifestyle. But then he told me his parents took him and his brother to Miami. Could it be that, like Jimmy, he told children fantastic tales, and the children believed them?

Pa wanted me to drive him to Bristol, to Halifax, and probably to Miami. I didn't take him to any of those places, although I probably should have. I have always felt bad about that. But I couldn't imagine being in a closed car for that long with a man who smelled as bad as a used open grave. Besides, what would we have talked about?

After Ma's death, I visited him alone one day at the senior unit, and we had one of the few serious conversations we ever had. We talked about his nephew Roger, whom he hoped would visit him. He said he needed new chair pads for the kitchen chairs before Roger came.

After more mundane conversations, I finally got up the courage to ask him if Ma had ever loved me. I could see he was stunned by my question. His head moved back in shock and he said, "Your mother loved you more than anything in the world."

I thought, *"What! Did I hear that right?"* Then I said, "Pa, she never told me."

He shook his head and said, "People don't go around telling each other that they love them."

It was a heartbreaking thing for him to have said to me. For a few seconds I stood in front of him. Ma had told me Pa had wanted me to be aborted, but I didn't know if that was true. I didn't think it was. I hoped it wasn't. I thought, *"This is the opportunity. Ask!"*

I wanted to ask him if he knew about Ma trying to kill me, but I finally decided not to do it. If I had asked him, there was no guarantee he would have told me the truth. Or maybe he hadn't known about it, and then he might have realized how much he had hurt her with his many lovers. Or maybe he would have said, "Yes." And I didn't know what I would have said in response to anything he would have said, so I didn't ask.

A short time later he was admitted to the hospital for heart issues. When I visited him, the doctor was cutting Pa's long, jagged toenails with tin snips. After the doctor left, Pa told me an orderly had put him in a whirlpool to ease his arthritis, but I suspect it was to clean him. They must have had to change the whirlpool water when they took him out.

It was clear to both Jimmy and me that he would not be returning to senior housing. He would have to go to a nursing home. There was no way I could have physically taken care of him, even if I wanted to. And I didn't.

We contacted the senior housing management, and we were told that we would have to remove all his things within two weeks or pay another month's rent.

We took the keys to the unit and opened it and were hit with the sweet smell of rotting food. The sink was full, past capacity, with dirty dishes. The stench was unbelievable. Jimmy started there, throwing the dishes into a garbage bag and cleaning the sink, as I opened all the windows and the door. We filled at least ten bags with garbage, food from the refrigerator, and filthy laundry that could not be cleaned. Jimmy put those bags and the by then broken kitchen chairs on the sidewalk outside the unit. I knew the garbage men would earn their money that week.

Ma and Pa had not lived in that unit long enough to justify wreaking such destruction. In a short time, they had done the same thing there as on Burnham Street and Till Street. Filthy white trash.

When Pa was discharged from the hospital, he called me and told me he was ready to go home. We had already cleaned out his senior unit, and I knew I could not physically take care of him if I brought him back to Till Street. I called his doctor, and he found a nursing home a few miles from the house. I felt bad about this. No one wants to end life in a nursing home, but I could see no other alternative.

When I visited him, I could see he was deteriorating fast. He was angry that he was in a nursing home. He couldn't do what he wanted to do or go where he wanted to go. The next time I saw him he was in bed. His eyes stared up at the ceiling and his pupils were like pinpoints. He said he thought he was dying, and that he wasn't afraid.

When I got home, I called his doctor, who admitted Pa to the hospital, to ICU. The last time I saw him at the hospital his heart was beating 170 beats per minute. I said, "Pa, I feel bad" and he answered, "Oh, don't feel bad." I sat there looking at him and I thought, *"I should tell him I love him, not because I care, but because that is what people are supposed to say when a*

137

parent is dying." I do not remember if I said it or not.

I went home, and the next morning around 5 AM the doctor called and told me he had died.

I thought the little amount of time when he was alone after Ma died, Pa was the happiest I ever saw him. He was making plans to do things. The two of them had a relationship of bondage, and in many ways, each ruined the other's life.

I buried Pa next to Ma in Bristol, RI. They had had a torturous life together, and mine had been intertwined with theirs in misery. I made sure they would rot in the ground next to each other.

I felt like my life had been a journey of walking a nightmarish road. The walk was over.

Weeks after Ma died, I cried about her death for less than five minutes because there never had been a relationship between us. I was sad that what could have been, never was. I mourned that void. When Pa died, I cried for a few minutes in front of his casket. We had made a small connection over the years, minuscule really. But I mourned that little semblance of a relationship.

That was in 1984. I didn't think much about them until 1988, when I learned about the healing power of forgiveness.

Chapter 9

Conception

Like most people, I cannot imagine my parents making love. I know they did, for I was born. Apart from the grossness of the mental image tied to that thought, I think the expression "making love" implies that there were at least some caring emotions between Ma and Pa. To be accurate, I should say I cannot imagine them having sex. But while my imagination refuses to consider this, I can draw conclusions about their sexual activities.

I suspect they were probably both drunk, or at least drinking. It would be unusual for one or the other, if not both, to have been sober. I cannot think of any reason why the occurrence of my conception would be any different.

I wonder why they had sex. Ma already knew that Pa was a serial adulterer. Had she no self-respect? Did she need him to continue to support her financially? Did she think if the sex was good, he would stop cheating on her? Did she love him? Did she just want sex? So many questions, but no answers.

I wonder how they could tolerate being intimate with each

other. Their standard of being clean consisted of washing in the bathroom sink with water heated on the kitchen stove. Ma tended to be cleaner than Pa, but not by much. I expect they had to hold their breath to tolerate the smell of the other. Also, to the best of my knowledge, neither of them used, or ever owned, a toothbrush.

I suspect those aspects of hygiene would not matter if drinking was involved. Or maybe the smell of stale beer or binge vomit overcame the other odors.

Eventually I know Ma and Pa, odors, filth, and drunkenness aside, had sex because I was born. Both of them impacted me as an embryo. I have seen people born with birth defects resulting from fetal alcohol syndrome. I considered myself fortunate to have been spared those lifelong burdens. I thought the 23 chromosomes from Pa must have been normal, as were the 23 from Ma. And I consider myself lucky in other ways.

Considering the number of sexual encounters Pa had, it surprises me that he didn't have gonorrhea or syphilis, which saved me from being born with the birth defects attributed to a sexually transmitted disease. During the time period of Pa's promiscuity, those were the two most common sexually transmitted diseases. Syphilis, at one time, was the most common cause of all miscarriages.[3] Congenital syphilis results

---

[3] Joseph Brown Cook. *Lippincott's Nursing Manuals: A Nurse's Handbook of Obstetrics.* Eighth edition, Revised and Reset, by Carolyn E. Gray and Mary Alberta Baker. Philadelphia: J.B. Lippincott, Company, 1917, 211.

in many more birth defects than gonorrhea, but the only ones that I recognized in myself were facial deformity and nervous systems disorders, and both of those could be accounted for by the amount they both drank. The main birth defect with gonorrhea is eye problems, including blindness; I clearly had not been infected with that. I am thankful that I had been spared the birth defects of a sexually transmitted disease.[4]

I am also fortunate to have been conceived in 1949 instead of in 2021, the year this memoir was published. With the frequent occurrence of many sexually transmitted diseases in 2021, it would be more likely that Pa would have contracted one, and I would have suffered the resulting birth defects. I am so thankful that AIDS did not exist at the time Pa was active. If he had caught that and infected Ma, I would have had it, too. Then I would have died from AIDS.

It does not seem that it would have been fair to me if I had escaped death by Ma's attempt at self-induced abortion only to die from a sexually transmitted disease given to me in my mother's womb. Beyond that, when considering his lifestyle, it is a surprise to me that he had either any desire for Ma or the ability to impregnate Ma. But, fortunately for me, he did.

This is how I think of my time in Ma's body. The half of me that came from Pa and the half of me that came from Ma, joined, and the cell which resulted can never be anything but

---

[4] See https://medlineplus.gov/ency/article/001344.htm for syphilis; general google.com search for gonorrhea on April 1, 2015.

me. I weighed 15 ten-millionths of a gram.[5]

That first day, I am one cell, then two, then four, and my cells continue to divide, becoming a more complete me, as I look for a safe place to grow in Ma's warm, nourishing, and safe womb. I continue to grow and develop with all sorts of fascinating things happening to me, until I turn four weeks old. Ma does not know about me.

By week 4, I am an embryo, and I grow quickly. I have the beginning of my brain, which has served me so well in my lifetime. In the next few weeks, I develop more of my body parts. My skeleton forms, my fingers and toes develop, I move on my own, my facial muscles develop, and I start to hiccup, frown, squint, furrow my brow, purse my lips, move my arms and legs, turn my head, touch my face, stretch, yawn, and suck. Ma begins to suspect that I am here.

Weeks 8 to 10 are great! I have a liver and kidneys, finger-prints and fingernails. I can bend my fingers as if there is an object in my palm, suck my thumb, and swallow, and I am sensitive to touch. I am in good shape! Ma knows I am here. I wish she would stop drinking and smoking. She seems to be doing both much more now.

In week 11, I start to practice breathing and I can urinate. I

---

[5] See "Fetal Development Week by Week," located online at www.babycenter.com/pregnancy-week-by-week/. See also the "Timeline Human Development: Embryology," located online at https://embryology.med.unsw.edu.au/embryology/index.php/Timel ine_human_development

smile. I smile when I urinate. Ma decides she wants to kill me. She talks to her father about how to do this. I don't know what the word "kill" means. But Ma says it so often about me that I assume it must be something special she wants to do for me because she loves me. With the thought of her love for me in my mind, I start to move around a lot when she drinks and smokes so she will know I want her to stop doing both. This doesn't work. In fact, every time I move, she drinks and smokes more.

And in week 12, anyone who had the technology and cared to look could see I am a girl. I have a distinctive face. I can kick, make a fist, turn my head, open my mouth, and press my lips together. I am now 3 inches long and weigh about 2 ounces. I am healthy. I can feel pain.

I suspect Ma didn't know about the pregnancy for quite a while. If she had realized it sooner, she would probably have found a way to kill me earlier in my development. Pregnancy tests were not available in the pharmacies back in 1949, so she had to wait until she had missed at least two periods to determine if she was pregnant. When she found out for sure, it probably took another week or more to decide what to do about me, and another week to decide to follow through with her plan to kill me.

Ma stopped this attempt to kill me, but only because she was afraid she would die, too. Her drinking and smoking were the least of the things I had to worry about; the chemical bath of death was a much more serious concern.

It is hard for me to imagine being inside of Ma, actually taking my life from her body, growing in what should have been her safe, warm, nourishing womb. It should have been a happy nine months for me with every beat of her heart loving me and bringing me what I needed to grow, from my one cell beginning to my complete full-term self.

As I got bigger and stronger, she got bigger too, and with each passing day, more filled with resentment.

But I am a strong embryo, with a will like steel. I have a picture of me in my mind's eye, hanging onto the inside of Ma's womb, supposedly a safe place – the safest place in the world to be for a baby.

I have already managed to hang on to her womb with my tiny fingernails and toenails, gripping her womb with all the power my little developing frame can muster, as she continued to drink and smoke. She didn't know I was here, and if she did, I doubt it would have stopped her consumption of either since she didn't want me. But I continue to hold on as beer, wine, and whiskey wash over me, bathing my tiny ears and nose and mouth; I imagine the nicotine making my tiny little lungs want to cough, although they don't know how to do it yet. Maybe I want to vomit from the combination of liquor and smoke, but I haven't developed enough to do that yet.

Then her father, my beloved Grandpa Herb, provides her with the 'medicine' that is supposed to force me to let go. Ma and her father hope I will be flushed out of her vagina like an unfortunate spontaneous abortion, down the toilet, through the drainpipe, into the sewer. But still I hang on. I will not let go, even though her bleeding starts. One by one my tiny toenails let go, first on one foot, then on the other. Both of my feet have lost their grip on Ma's womb. I am still hanging on to the wall, but it is getting wet and slippery, and only my fingernails keep me from certain death. One by one by one by one by one, the fingernails on my left hand let go of her womb. I have only five fingernails left to hold on with, and I am getting weak and tired. Finally, only one fingernail is still clinging to her womb, but I hang on with a strong death grip. I hang on through more days until the impact of the murderous medicine passes.

I think now of what would have happened if I had just let go with that last fingernail, too weak to hang onto the slippery wall anymore. I wonder if I thought, *I am bruised and defeated; just let go.* But then, no! I bend my tiny finger at the first and second joint, digging my fingernail further into my mother's flesh. I feel her whole body involuntarily flinch, and she puts her hands on her belly. Then I think, *"What is this? Blood?" I hope the wall doesn't get more slippery. I can't hang on much longer. Hey, Ma! I'm not going anywhere. I'm holding on. If I die, you die!*

If I had let go, I would have been flushed out of Ma, an eliminated, 3-inch clump of tissue and cells. I would never have loved Jimmy or Bill, had a family with grandchildren or great-grandchildren. I would never have heard Kid Rock sing at the Super Bowl, nor seen the Broadway show *CATS!*, nor enjoyed an Irish coffee in Waterford, Ireland. I would never have been Catholic. My only consolation is, once conceived, I would have continued on as me forever.

But I hung on. Ma started to bleed more from the puncture wound I put in the wall of her womb. Her fear of death saved me, and when she saw the soaking and then the gushes of bright red blood, she feared that the medicine she was taking to kill me would lead to her own death as well. And so, she stopped taking it. We both lived. My tiny fingernails and toenails, and my iron will, saved us both.

In my mind's eye, I see the womb wall slowly becoming easier to hang onto – one by one I am able to hold on with two fingers, then another, and finally my toes. And I hang on for dear life.

Ma was a selfish woman who didn't want to wait nine months for me to be born. She could have given me up for adoption or left me with a social service agency. Perhaps I would have been adopted into a happy family that would have loved me.

She kept me due to pride. Her pride kept her from divorcing my cheating father, and her pride wouldn't let her face people asking where her missing baby was.

I wonder what she thought about when my presence made her want to vomit? What she felt when I started moving around? What she thought when I started kicking her belly? Or what she imagined when I was ready to come out and greet the world, a new life.

I was born in 1950. Approximately eleven years later, Ma told me she had tried to kill me.

Since then, I have been hanging on.

My first husband, Jimmy, a devout Catholic who would never miss Sunday Mass, came home one Sunday just before Christmas, and told me about a disturbing homily he had heard at Mass that day. At the time, Jimmy did not know I was an abortion survivor. In fact, I never thought of myself as one until years later when I told my life story to a coworker. My coworker looked at me and said the words, "You are an abortion survivor." I thought of abortion survivors as infants who were forced from the womb in unsuccessful attempts to kill them. I had remained in Ma's womb, saved by her fear of her own death.

The homily that disturbed Jimmy so much that Sunday was a pro-life one. In it, a baby talks to herself within her mother's womb. On the day of her conception, she says, "They are going to be so excited when they find out I am here. I can't wait till the day they find out. They will be so happy, so eager to welcome me into their lives and make a family."

About six weeks later, the baby says, "She found out today! My mother found out that I am here, and she is going to be a mother. She is so happy she started to cry when the doctor told her the news. She is going to tell my father tonight. I am so excited! The doctor told her that her due date is in November.

I will be here for Christmas. I wonder what they will give me? I bet they will shower me with love and gifts! How exciting! When Mom told Dad she is going to have me, he was so overcome with joy he sat at the table and put his head in his hands. He asked Mom, 'What do you want to do?' She started crying and said, 'You know.'"

The baby continued, "How great! He wants to know what she wants to get me for Christmas, and she thinks he already knows!"

The homily continued, relating the events of another month of pregnancy, with the baby's happy anticipation of its birth and first Christmas.

At the end of the homily, the baby says, "I can't believe it. I'm not going to have a first Christmas. My parents killed me today. They killed me. They actually didn't love me at all."

I remember when Jimmy told me about this homily, I felt a smothering blanket of sadness descend on me. My chest felt heavy, and I had trouble getting air in and out of my lungs. I wanted to cry but was so distraught I could not shed one tear. It felt as if my soul was crying, wailing, screaming, and my body could only listen in deep silence. At the time, I considered myself a pro-choice feminist, and suddenly I became aware of what pro-choice meant. The homily made abortion a personal issue for me. Hearing Jimmy relate it changed my perspective from an outward-looking one focusing on Ma – *my mother* tried to kill me – to an inward-looking one – my mother tried to kill *me*. I knew embryos did not wonder what gifts they would receive at Christmas any more than I hung onto the wall of my mother's womb with my fingernails and toenails, saving my life by making a puncture wound. But that subtle change in emphasis changed me. I realized the possibility of my death, of not being, in a way I had not realized it before. I felt a sadness that I imagine bordered on the oppression of the grave. I had almost not been born. And I would not even have had a grave. Instead, in the sewer, I might have been lunch for mangy rats. And I was not even big enough to satisfy their hunger.

When Jimmy told me about the homily, I already knew, for decades, the story of Ma's pregnancy and her attempt to kill me. I never could forget that monologue.

Ma sat me down in a kitchen chair to the left of the chrome and Formica table. I was in front of the kitchen window, and I seem to remember I could only see black when I looked through the window so it must have been early evening or nighttime. Ma said she had an important story to tell me. I remember she looked serious. She didn't smile, but that was not unusual; she rarely smiled. The expression in her brown eyes was cold and angry. Even her voice sounded different from the way it usually did. Instead of being slurred from one beer or wine too many, or shrill with anger, it sounded crisp and hard, with an edge to it. Her body movements looked stiff and rigid, as if she had turned into a robot. When I think back to that most important day of my life, and the story she told me that changed my perspective on the world, I remember her being intense. I could see her struggling to get the words exactly right. Now when I recall that memory, I think that she looked like a bomb squad policewoman approaching a live explosive.

The story was a simple one. At forty, she thought she was starting the change. Her voice was cold and distant, but I didn't know why. Her facial expression and movement signaled the importance of the story. She explained she had bad arthritis, and the doctor had given her some medicine to help reduce the pain and make her joints work as they should. But, she said, he didn't tell her one of the side effects of the drug was increased fertility. At 40, she went on the drug and at 41 she had me. Then she looked at me like I should know what that meant.

If the story had ended there, I would have thought it just another strange encounter with Ma, of which there were too many. But she went on. She told me she didn't want to be pregnant, so she went to her father – whom I had adored prior to hearing this story – and told him of her pregnancy and her wish to end it. She said she asked him what she could do. He went out, she said, and found a pharmacist who gave her some medicine to take. She took it and shortly thereafter, started to bleed. The blood scared her. She was afraid she might die, so she stopped taking the medicine. When the bleeding stopped, she was still pregnant and thus, months later, I was born.

I was just 11 years old when Ma told me she had tried to kill me. To the best of my knowledge, I was her only pregnancy. I didn't have the words to express it then, as I was just a little girl, but I never cared about her again. She told me the story, and I turned off my love like the light leaving a room when someone flips off the switch. I had thought that they loved me the way I loved them – Ma, Pa, my grandfather. It had never occurred to me that they saw me as an unwanted inconvenience. I felt devastated, and I remained that way for decades.

I have often wondered why Ma told me that story. If she had never told me, I would have continued loving her. Looking back, I suspect she wanted a confidant. Maybe she thought it would bring us closer. She and I behaved more like friends for years, and as her own friends and family visited her less frequently every year, I think she wanted us to bond more closely. In fairness to her, I don't think she knew this would be the turning point in our relationship. She crossed a boundary that could never be uncrossed when she told me she tried to kill me. I went from loving her to hating her, and as I grew up, to thinking of her as an irrelevant nuisance that I was forced to deal with.

Regardless of the situation of my conception and survival, I came into this world by Cesarean in March 1950. Ma told me she didn't want to go through labor. She said she feared the pain and told me she would "look at herself and wonder how that big thing could come out of her." After talking to Dr. Rivas, he agreed she could have a Cesarean.

When I was about twelve, Ma and Pa told me about that experience. Pa told me that the winter of 1949-1950 was a tough one. He said when there was a snow or ice storm, or the temperatures went below freezing, he would go outside every hour or so to start the car in case Ma needed to go to the hospital. I thought it was a nice thing for a husband to do for his wife and for a father to do for his daughter. This conversation led me to consider them as a husband and wife, rather than as just Ma and Pa. They had a life apart from me, and my realizing that helped me see the life the three of us lived together in a different context.

And then Ma told me that after the surgery, when the anesthesia wore off, the nurse came into her room bringing me to her. Ma said she held me close and said, "I am going to give you such a beautiful home." When she told me that, I wondered if the morphine had been talking or if she cared for me just a little bit. I still wonder.

Chapter 10

The Times

As I grew up, I had a lot of questions about Ma's attempt to kill me. What was the social and legal environment in 1949 and 1950 concerning abortion? What drugs were available for Ma to take when she decided to kill me? What were the possible birth defects that I had, or had escaped having, from those drugs? Or from her continued smoking and drinking, both behaviors that are now recognized as risky, but in the 1940s were not? Or from Pa's promiscuity? What impact did Ma's decision to tell me about the abortion attempt have on my personality? All serious questions. I wasn't sure I would be able to find the answers, but I knew I had to try. And fortunately, as an academic, I knew how to do the research.

A Short History of Abortion in the United States

I wanted to better understand what Ma would have faced when she decided to kill me. I knew abortion was illegal at the time, but I also knew that illegality did not mean there was no access to abortion services. I assumed that an abortion would be difficult to procure and a rare occurrence.

By 1949, World War II had ended, most of the troops had returned from Europe and Asia, and women were returning to their homes instead of working outside of them. Looking back on the decade that began in 1950, I think most people saw it as a time of making homes and families, a golden age of America that focused on the family. Five days a week, husbands left the home to work, wives stayed home and took care of the house and the family, children went to school and obediently learned their lessons. At night, the family would eat a delicious meal created by the wife, and after she cleaned the kitchen, she would join everyone already sitting in the parlor playing board games or watching television. On weekends, everyone would go to religious services, visit relatives, and have s special dinner.

But I wondered, being realistic, was life really ever like that?

I am sure that at least some Americans did live that kind of life, others thought they should but didn't, and still others revolted against it. Perhaps many of the last group were women who wanted to limit the number of children they had so they could live life as they saw fit. At least some, if not many, of those women must have turned to abortion.

The social and political climate surrounding abortion in 1949, and the decades prior to Roe v. Wade, was based on centuries of development. This development is summarized by Suzanne Staggenborg, a sociologist whose primary work is done in the area of social movements.[6]

The states were originally guided on the matter of abortion by British common law, which permitted abortion until 'quickening,' the point about midway through pregnancy when the woman first perceives fetal movement. Although abortion before quickening was socially acceptable and there was no grass-roots anti-abortion movement before the twentieth century, there was a successful campaign to outlaw abortion in the nineteenth century that was initiated not by religious leaders - as might be expected - but by physicians. The physicians who led this campaign were 'regular' doctors motivated in large part by their desire to regulate medicine and to drive out the 'irregular' doctors who were most likely to perform abortions. The power of these regular physicians grew with the formation of the American Medical Association (AMA) in 1845 and later from a political alliance with the anti-obscenity movement led by Anthony Comstock in the 1870s. But because there was no popular movement to resist the pressure exerted by the AMA and its members, by 1900 abortion had been outlawed by every state in the nation.

---

[6] Suzanne Staggenborg, *The Pro-Choice Movement: Organization and Activism in the Abortion Conflict*. New York: Oxford University Press, 1991, 3. She cites James Mohr, *Abortion in America: The Origins and Evolution of National Policy*, Oxford University Press, 1979.

This illegality resulted in two categories of abortion: therapeutic and illegal. Doctors performed therapeutic abortions for medical and psychiatric reasons that were for the health of the woman and were legal. Mark Graber, an expert in constitutional law, states that most of these abortions were performed on affluent white women, although rates per live births varied considerably from hospital to hospital and from state to state.[7]

Illegal abortions contained two subcategories; criminal abortions, those performed by another person on a pregnant woman, and self-induced abortions, or those performed by the pregnant woman on herself. Criminal abortionists, as described by Graber, were "Not subject to state regulation and inspection...Many women had little choice as to who would terminate their pregnancy. Lucky women had their abortions clandestinely terminated by licensed doctors in medical settings; unlucky women might find themselves aborted by a mechanic in the back of a car."[8]

Graber quotes, "'A large number of illegal abortions...were self-induced or performed by unskilled and untrained

---

[7] Mark Graber, Rethinking Abortion: Equal Choice, the Constitution, and Reproductive Politics. Princeton, NJ: Princeton University Press, 1996, 50-51.

[8] Graber, 60.

personnel working under dangerous septic conditions, unaccountable to professional guidelines and safeguards and unreached by ordinary government licensing procedures or others safeguards.'"[9]

Anecdotal evidence shows that illegal abortions were not difficult to obtain for the wealthy. Graber quotes an interesting statement. "Garrett Hardin, a leading authority on population control, stated that 'in California, it is safe to say that any knowledgeable woman with $500 in her pocket can secure an abortion.'"[10] That amount of money would have been huge in the time prior to Roe v. Wade, so many women chose other means to abort.

Self-induced abortions were relegated to desperate women, those who did not have enough money to pay for an abortion by a professional or who did not have access to a network that would send the woman to an abortionist. Other women may have preferred self-induced abortion, based on herbal knowledge handed down from mother to daughter, or for privacy within the home.

Determining the number of annual abortions prior to Roe V. Wade is difficult because only therapeutic abortions were controlled and thus recorded, and even therapeutic abortion statistics are not readily available. Graber cites some statistics:

Access to legal abortions before *Roe* differed significantly

---

[9] Graber, 63.

[10] Graber, 60.

in jurisdictions that adopted the same legal language. In the late 1960s, California, Maryland, Colorado, Virginia, South Carolina, and North Carolina passed nearly identical reform measures based on the recommendations of the American Law Institute (ALI). The respective legal abortion rates in these states in 1970, however, were 135, 102, 41, 13, 7, and 7 per thousand live births. [11]

My interest is in the number and causes of non-therapeutic abortions. Graber stated that some "scholars estimate one in every three to five pregnancies was aborted in the first seventy years of the twentieth century. During the 1950s and 1960s, close to one million illegal abortions were performed every year. Some public health specialists suggest that as many as two to three million abortions were performed annually in the United States during the early twentieth century."[12] Other estimates, based on birth rates, range from 200,000 to 1.3 million per year.[13]

Rickie Solinger, a historian concerned with reproductive

---

[11] Graber, 42.

[12] See Graber, Chapter II, endnotes 19 and 20.

[13] See Russell S. Fisher, "Criminal Abortion," Journal of Criminal Law and Criminology 42:2, July-August 1951 accessed scholarlycommons.law.northwestern.edu/jclc, p. 242 (note that Taussig, who calculated the lower figure cited by Fisher, eventually stated his calculations were incorrect.); Heather D. Boonstra, Rachel Benson Gold, Cory L. Richards, and Lawrence F. Finer, *Abortion In Women's Lives*, Guttmacher Institute, 2006, Chapter 2.

rights, summarized the data, saying, "The truth is that even when blocked by laws, institutions, and authorities, up to one million women a year sought and obtained abortions in the illegal era – though not without a struggle."[14]

So, what drugs were available in 1949?

Specifically, my interest is in self-induced abortions because that was how Ma had attempted to kill me. I found information about a large number of herbs and drugs available on the market in 1949 that could cause an abortion.[15] These

---

[14] Rickie Solinger, "Pregnancy and Power before Roe V. Wade, 1950-1970," in Rickie Solinger (ed), *Abortion Wars: A Half Century of Struggle, 1950-2000*. London: University of California Press, 1998, 16.

[15] Fisher noted there were other methods of abortion commonly used, including surgery, vaginal douching, vaginal creams (p. 242). See also *A Nurse's Handbook of Obstetrics*, where reference is made to some of these herbs and medicines, as well as to douches, as causing miscarriage. Pregnant women often suffer from constipation or diarrhea. In the case of constipation, a warning is given: "Castor oil or aloes must of course not be used." Further on in the *Handbook*, diarrhea is mentioned as a danger to the baby. "Prolonged or severe diarrhea is often a direct cause of miscarriage ..." Later in the *Handbook*, more time is spent on constipation and diarrhea.

"Diarrhea occasionally occurs during pregnancy, and its onset should be reported at once to the medical attendant. If it is allowed to persist it may result in a miscarriage, either because

could be categorized as purgatives that caused bowel evacuation (castor oil, croton oil, aloes); intestinal and pelvic irritants (oils of pennyroyal, tansy, savin, and rue); stimulants that cause uterine muscle contractions (quinine, ergot, pituitary extract); and systematic poisons taken by mouth (lead salts, kerosene, apiol, mercury salts, oil of wintergreen, nitrobenzene).

When I began my research, I looked for a liquid Ma could have drunk, as she told me that was what she had done. I assumed it was a liquid in the fourth category, chemicals that were systemic poisons. People thought the baby would die and the mother would live because the dose of poison would be greater for the baby than for the mother. This often did not happen and sometimes both the baby and the mother died. Ma probably sensed that. I concluded that she probably took a prescription or herbal medicine that the pharmacist gave my grandfather. Ma would have been looking for something that would kill me but be very safe for her to take. I thought she probably took a stimulant that would cause uterine contrac-

---

of the severe straining efforts at stool or on account of an extension of the existing intestinal inflammation. Castor oil, so commonly given at the onset of a simple diarrhea, cannot be allowed during pregnancy. The drugs are so well-marked that they have earned for it the unenviable name of 'the poor woman's ergot.'

tions, perhaps quinine pills.[16] Then I discovered that quinine liquid with cocoa – to mask the quinine taste – was available at the time. I assumed that was the abortifacient she took, but I am aware that I will never know with certainty.

The psychological effects of finding out I was an abortion survivor were much worse than the physical ones. In a literature search, I discovered material about abortion survivor guilt (children who know their mother aborted one of their siblings); guilt of the woman who had the abortion; guilt of the father who was in favor of the abortion; and lastly, and somewhat applicable to me, the effects on the unwanted child when the mother was denied abortion.

In this last category of studies, children born between 1961 and 1963 to women in Prague who were denied an abortion

---

[16] A friend put me in contact with Dr. Imre Teglasy of Hungary. His mother tried to abort him using quinine pills. His story, which mirrors mine in many ways, led me to consider quinine as the possible abortifacient Ma used.

In Lippincott, 211, the author describes the dilemma a doctor is faced with when a pregnant woman has malaria. He said, "Malaria is very apt to cause abortion, either by reason of its high temperature or because of the large doses of quinine given for its control...the physician is between two horns of a dilemma when he encounters severe malaria complicating pregnancy, for if quinine is not given, through fear of causing miscarriage, the high temperature of the disease will most probably do so."

twice were compared with babies born of mothers pair-matched for socioeconomic status and husband's (or partner's) presence in the home. In the section, *Interpreting the Findings*, the authors of one study said,

> Unwantedness in early pregnancy foreshadows a family atmosphere unlikely to be conducive to healthy child-rearing. ...an alternative interpretation of the study results may be in terms of parental preoccupation, a term used... to describe mothers who are physically present but psychologically absent. Preoccupation encompasses a broad range of parental behavior and vagaries in limit setting. It is questionable however, whether parental preoccupation or environmental deprivation alone can explain differences observed in early medical records.[17]

So, what birth defects occurred from smoking and drinking? For much of my life, I assumed the physical problems I have – a head too small for my body, facial abnormalities, joint issues on the left side of my body – were side effects of the abortifacient Ma took. While doing research, I discovered the birth defects that result when a woman drinks during preg-

---

[17] Henry P. David. "Born Unwanted: Mental Health Costs and Consequences,"*American Journal of Orthopsychiatry* 81:2 2011, 190. See also, Henry P. David, "Born Unwanted: Long-Term Developmental Effects of Denied Abortion," *Journal of Social Issues* 48:3 1992, 163-181.

nancy.

Ma continued to drink and smoke while she was pregnant with me. I would not be surprised if the frequency with which she did both increased once she learned of the pregnancy as she experienced more stress while deciding whether or not to kill me. Then, once she decided to stop taking the abortifacient, she probably continued to drink and smoke frequently because of the stress of having an unwanted baby. In the interests of justice, I have to say that I do not think Ma drank and smoked to hurt me. I don't believe she, or anyone else in that time period, realized the effects these chemicals would have on an unborn child.

According to the Center for Disease Control Fact Sheet,[18] there is no safe amount of any kind of alcohol a pregnant woman, or one who is trying to become pregnant, can consume. When a pregnant woman drinks, the alcohol enters the baby through the umbilical cord. This can result in birth defects that last for the life of the person.

There exist many signs and symptoms of fetal alcohol spectrum disorders. The ones that I recognize in myself are small head size, poor coordination, delayed language ability, and abnormal facial features.

Jimmy looked at the size of my head and decided that my

---

[18] CDC Fact Sheet on FASD, found at http://www.cdc.gov/ncbddd/fasd/facts.html and CDC Fact Sheet on Smoking and Pregnancy, found at http://www.cdc.gov/reproductivehealth/tobaccousepregnancy/

nickname should be Pinhead. He said that word accurately described my head size. There is no question that my head is too small for my body. I fit in child-sized hats, and sometimes they are loose. When I participate in a graduation ceremony, I have to order the smallest size cap, and then I have to use bobby pins to keep it on.

When I was in my teens, I was walking home from high school one day when I heard a boy across the street yell at me, "For crying out loud, learn how to walk." I wondered what he was talking about until I realized he had noticed my unusual gait. As an adult, a professor, I once heard one of my students say he had noticed me hobbling to class. *Hobbling?* How insulting! One day I was walking through an audience to reach the stage to give a presentation, when I partially lost my balance. A woman asked me, "Are you all right?" I thought to myself, *"Yes, lady, I do these pirouettes routinely as I try to remain standing. I have many other spontaneous hip, knee, and ankle movements if you would like to see them for your amusement."* Sometimes, I am so uncoordinated that I feel like a marionette whose strings are being manipulated by a drunk. Years ago, I told my husband I would open a door for him, as he was carrying a heavy box. I lurched for the door, turned in a semi-circle, and missed the handle. The problems continue.

Pa asked me once if I would like to hear the situation surrounding both my first walk and my first word. Mildly curious, I said yes. I thought I might have tried to stand up and might have said, "Ma." But Pa said he was out in the backyard doing some work and had brought me outside to enjoy the air. I was sitting on the ground, and he was a good distance away from me. He said I suddenly stood up, started running towards him, and screamed "fishbath." I have to admit I was not convinced that Pa was telling the truth, but when I asked Ma, she said yes, what he had said was true. After hearing her say that, I wondered if they were both lying. Really, who says fishbath?

In further investigation of FASD, I used the National Organization on Fetal Alcohol Syndrome website.[19] This organization listed additional symptoms, including a thin upper lip, underdeveloped jaw, and small eye openings. I recognize all of these in myself.

And lastly, a quick Google search resulted in sites that also mention issues with social skills, social communication problems, sensory processing, spina bifida, and joint anomalies, most of which I recognize in myself. I was never diagnosed with spina bifida, but my osteoporosis doctor told me I almost had it.

I was born with an unusual face. My lower jaw was set back on my face, and my upper jaw protruded far out from my face. My upper lip is very thin, and my eye openings are small. My face was, in my opinion, hideous. And it was placed on the front of a head that was too small. I often think, *"At least it wasn't placed on the side of my head."*

---

[19] The National Organization on Fetal Alcohol Syndrome website is http://www.nofas.org/

One day I was in the car with Jimmy, stopped at a red light, when he saw a man who could have been my twin before I had facial surgery. Jimmy said, "Whoa. That is one weird looking guy." I recognized that man's face as looking like mine before I had it surgically altered. I wanted to jump out of the car and tell this stranger that I once looked like he did and that he could be fixed like I had been.

But I didn't. The light turned green, and Jimmy drove on. As we left, I noticed the man walked with the same gait as me. I prayed, "Dear God in Heaven, please help that poor man. Give him strength and self-confidence and lead him to a capable surgeon."

The worst part of my face was the lower half. I eventually had extensive orthodontic work done (twice, 30 years apart) by an orthodontist who specialized in working with adults. Then I had surgery at a major New England dental school. The surgeon sliced through both sides of my jaw vertically and pulled the jaw down and forward. He reattached the jaw with wires, and I believe he said screws. I recovered, jaw wired shut for weeks. I believe that after the surgery to repair the lower part of my face, my jawline, the area below my eyes and the tip of my nose, and my upper mouth, I looked almost normal.

Once I had healed, I received three orthodontic appliances that I am to wear until I die. One is permanently attached behind my bottom front teeth. One I wear on my bottom teeth for a few hours each night to hold my jaw forward. When I take that appliance out, I put in an appliance that keeps my top teeth back. I wear this one all night. For almost four decades now, I have followed the rules given to me by the surgeon and orthodontist.

Today, my chin clearly juts to the left, and recently my jaw has stopped working correctly. If I open my mouth wide, my jaw shoots down and moves to the left, as if Howdy Doody's jaw has decided to detach and go for a walk. Thanks Ma.

Fortunately, I can disguise my thin upper lip with lip liner applied outside of my lip line.

And I can also disguise my small eye openings with eyeliner, concealer, two shades of eye shadow, and mascara.

Another two related symptoms of FASD are spina bifida and joint anomalies. When I started going to a doctor for osteoporosis, he told me that I had almost had spina bifida. I also learned that the joints on the left side of my body are not the same size as those on the right side. "Thank you, God," I pray, "for sparing me from spina bifida."

The FASD-related symptoms have to do with social skills, social communication problems, and sensory processing. I am a solitary person. I enjoy social interaction with family, friends, and coworkers, but only for a limited amount of time and in one-on-one situations. The only exception to this is when I am in a position of authority, like a professor in a classroom or a presenter at a conference. In those circumstances, I think of the group I am addressing as one person, not as a collection of individuals.

When I teach a class or present a paper, I work the crowd.

I convey information in a casual, almost conversational, tone. I tell appropriate jokes and stories, and I act friendly and open. Inside, I feel like I am on stage. The first large group I addressed, of over 300 people, went well. Some people in the audience thought I was addressing just them. I was. I was addressing 300 people as one entity.

Unfortunately, I cannot always be the person who does the addressing, and that is when I realize how weird it is to be solitary. In a conversation with three or four people, I usually say almost nothing, overwhelmed by the amount of conversation, the ebb and flow of it, the rhythm. I cannot see a place to enter into it, a space I can step into. I have been told this makes people think I am unfriendly or conceited.

Of course, it is dangerous for someone who is not a medical doctor, or even for someone who is, to self-diagnose. I do not know if I officially fit on the Fetal Alcohol Spectrum Disorder, but I recognize many of the markers as things I have struggled with throughout my life.

I prefer to think that the issues I have trace back to Ma drinking during her pregnancy, and not to the abortifacient she took. When Ma drank, she probably had no idea it would hurt me, but Ma took the abortifacient to kill me. It is easier for me to live with the first option than the second one. The first seems more forgivable, the second, less so. But that does not mean I am correct. My defects could be caused by the drinking and the smoking, or the abortifacient she drank, or the combination of the two.

I think of how lucky I am that Ma wasn't born decades later. If she lived now, and tried to abort me, I would have died due to the new and effective methods of terminating pregnancies.

Chapter 11

On Forgiveness

Ma and Pa died when I was 34. After the funerals, the paperwork, and the decisions on what to do with their material possessions, I rarely thought about them for almost four years. Our relationship had been contentious, and in many ways, I felt glad it was over. I did not miss Ma screaming at me or at Pa, or her daily reminders to Pa about his infidelities. I did not miss her frequent accusations to me that I had ruined her life. Nor did I miss Pa, who was the cause of all her anger and frustration.

She reminded me so often that I had ruined her life that I became immune to the accusation. I had been born, and so her life was ruined. But I knew I was born because she feared dying. That wasn't my fault, but hers. My life became so much more peaceful without their presence, either in my house or in my life. I learned to love the sound of silence; the beautiful sound of non-screaming, of non-arguing. God, I loved the quiet. I could almost breathe it in.

Peace. Finally, peace because they were in their graves.

Well, peace for a while anyway.

I remember reading something about peace not being just a state of non-war. We all know there is war and there is peace. But there is also a state where war has ended, but peace – order, reconciliation, solidarity – has not yet occurred. That in-between state is non-war. The battles are over, but the resentment, hatred, and desire for revenge remain with victor and vanquished. That is not peace.

What I experienced after Ma and Pa died was a state of non-war. Ma had been at war with me since my conception and with Pa since before the first anniversary of their wedding day. Now that they were dead, I had non-war, which I enjoyed enormously. I didn't know that I had not yet achieved peace. I mistook non-war for the state I desired.

Four years after Ma and Pa died, Jimmy and I took a family trip to Rome. Included in our group were Jimmy's mother and other family members. We had asked his mother what she wanted to do for her 75th birthday, and she had quickly said, "Go to Rome."

Jimmy and his mother were devout Catholics, and to some extent, the other members of his family practiced Catholicism. While in Rome, Jimmy and his family, without me, went to one of John Paul II's Wednesday audiences. After the event, his mother told Jimmy that it had been the most important day of her life, more important than the day she got married or the days she had her children. I remember thinking, *"Oh brother.*

You have got to be kidding."

I could not understand the extent of their devotion and piety. I was neither Catholic nor devout. I had nothing against Catholicism; I just considered it, and all religion, as irrelevant.

The only reason I agreed to go to Rome with the family was that Jimmy and I had a discussion, while still in Connecticut, about how the trip would be managed. We agreed that every day all of us would have breakfast together. Then Jimmy and the family would go to religious sites, and I would go shopping, see the ancient ruins, or visit a museum. At the end of the day, we would meet and have dinner together. This arrangement worked for eight days.

A few nights later, after dinner, Jimmy asked me if we could all do something together as a family. I reminded him that we were already eating breakfast and dinner together. He suggested that we all go on a bus tour. I reminded him that we had agreed we would only have breakfast and dinner together. He said it would mean a lot to him if we all spent a day together in Rome. I reminded him that I did not think it would be a good way to spend any day, especially a day in Rome. I finally agreed to consider it since he was paying for the trip.

I thought about my plan to buy a red leather handbag the next day and realized I would have to forgo it if I went on a tour. I knew that pocketbook would bring me a lot more happiness than his tour.

I snarled, "Okay."

I agreed to go on a family tour if he could find one that had nothing religious on the itinerary. I assumed I had given him an impossible task, but I had not. He went to get a tour brochure at the hotel desk and in it, he found one tour that went outside of Rome and visited only one religious site. He asked me if I would go and added that I could wait in the bus while the rest of the family visited the religious site. "Alright," I snarled, with just a little more anger in my voice. I promised myself he would pay for this when we returned to the States.

After breakfast the next day, we all boarded the bus for the trip outside of the walls. I wasn't on the bus long before I noticed that it had neither air conditioning nor a toilet. When we got to the catacombs, the one religious site on the tour, I had the choice of waiting in an overheated metal box for the family to return, or to go on the tour. I chose the catacombs.

I rushed through the area where a priest was offering Mass, wondering why so many people were attending Mass when it was not Sunday. I searched for the group and joined them as they went to the place the tour guide was to meet us. I thought I would be able to wander around alone, but I was told I could not because people sometimes got lost in the underground passageways. As a group, we walked down the dark and dank passages, passing the graves of people dead so long I imagined they were by now only dust. Finally, we entered a small opening, almost a room, with a table in the middle. At one point the table was an altar or was supposed to represent one. I looked around and wondered why this was a tourist attraction. It was a barren place, underground.

Underground, in an ancient cemetery, in a room that used to function as a church. To me, a non-believer, it was an odd place to find myself.

The tour guide was a slender Asian priest, dressed in an immaculate black outfit that looked like a formal dress. I later learned it was called a cassock. He stood, not at what would be the head of the table, but on the longer side, as if the table was an altar. Everyone crowded into the room, which was not large enough to accommodate a busload of tourists. I could smell sunscreen, body odor, and sweat. I stood directly across from the priest, so close to the table that I could feel the front of my legs lightly pressed against it.

By a combination of the force of his silence and his expectant posture, the priest commanded the attention of everyone in the room. Including me.

He told us the story of the catacombs and some of the people who were buried there. I did not think he was trying to evangelize the people in the group – he probably thought people would not visit the catacombs if they were not Christian – but was trying to tell us the history of the place. Overall, I do not remember what he said in the approximately five minutes that he talked, although I remember him mentioning virgins and martyrs. I thought, *"Always with the virgins. What is it about Catholics and their issues with sex?"*

While I stood listening to this quiet-spoken man, who had just the slightest hint of an Asian accent, perhaps Vietnamese,

I felt as if time stood still in that room, or no longer existed, or perhaps didn't matter. It was as if, for just an instant in my life, the eternal and present coincided where I stood, and I could see history in my mind's eye, the then and the now, and perhaps even a little bit of the future. I could sense the *then* of Jesus' life and the belief of the people in the catacombs and the *now* of my life as it confronted a reality new to me, and the *future* of the continued effects of that life lived on Earth 2000 years ago. I could feel my heart beat very slowly in my chest, the sound echoing in my ears as if I was hearing my footsteps walk down the hallway to eternity. And I could see, with my mind's eye, a clarity that I had never had before, nor after. I saw the words "The Truth is found in the Catholic Church." I remember "Truth" not "truth." The first letter of "Truth" was capitalized; it was not "truth." At the time I had no idea that Truth referred to Jesus. I learned that later.

I responded because I knew the experience came from an external source. I knew it was not from my imagination - but from someone who could make me see a sentence in my mind as clear a typed line, with a message of eternal importance.

And I decided in much less than five seconds, most likely between one heartbeat and the next, that I had to convert. I would have despaired if I had not immediately made the choice once it was offered to me.

My conversion was a dramatic intellectual one. The door to a place I had never believed in, nor seen, opened, and I sensed the joy beyond it.

The priest stopped talking. We walked out of the opening, and followed him through the passageways, by the graves of people who were holy dust mixed with the dust of the grave. We continued on our way. No one could see that I was no longer the same me who had entered the catacombs a little while before, not even my family. The old me was gone, and the transforming process had begun, which continues to this day.

We finished the tour, went back to the hotel, had dinner, packed, slept, took the bus to the airport, boarded the plane, flew home, picked up our car, and drove home. I pondered my experience in silence during all those activities.

A few days later, after we had gotten back into our daily routine, I asked Jimmy to make an appointment with his priest because I wanted to become Catholic. He laughed as if I had just told him a joke. At the time, I was politically liberal and had strong secular humanist leanings. It did not surprise me that he didn't believe me. In fact, he thought I was making fun of him and his piety. I finally convinced him, and Jimmy made the appointment.

Fr. Stan and I agreed to meet at 10:00 AM every Saturday morning, and for many months we did. I quickly moved beyond the basics of the faith and started reading theological works from his library. I studied with him every Saturday, and we discussed things as varied as how God can be one and three, what the hypostatic union is, whether Mary is really Mediatrix, what the phrase "the Body of Christ" means, what happened at

Vatican Council II, and original sin. I have never studied so intently or passionately as I did with him. I studied for so long that one morning when I knocked on the rectory door, the housekeeper looked at me with pity and said, "You're having a lot of trouble learning this, aren't you, dear?" I just smiled.

After a year of studying with Fr. Stan, I became Catholic before an evening liturgy on February 22, 1988.

The interesting thing about Catholicism is that it is not just about external activity – like going to Mass, receiving the sacraments, and getting buried in a certain cemetery – but about internal changes. One day, I realized what I was saying when I recited the Our Father prayer, "Forgive us our trespasses as we forgive those who trespass against us." I knew I had to forgive Ma, most of all, for trying to kill me and for telling me about the attempt. I had to forgive Ma and Pa for our lack of relationship, for their neglect of me as a child, for their verbal and psychological abuse of me, and for their abuse of each other. I had to forgive myself for retaliating against them for the things they had done to me over the years. And I had to forgive Jimmy for asking my parents to leave the house on Till Street, and again to forgive myself for the resentment I had felt against him for putting me in such an awkward position.

Then I remembered that Jesus died on the Cross to pay the price for my sins, to forgive me so that I could attain Heaven and spend eternity there. If Jesus could forgive me, how could

I not forgive them.

I started to think about the commandment to honor your father and mother. How do you honor, respect, or love people like Ma and Pa? They were merciless. But so was I. They had hurt me more times than I could remember. I carried the physical scars of my unpleasant gestation, and more psychological abuse and neglect than I could ever record in a memoir. As an adult, I remembered those things, and although I didn't often lash back at them, when I did, I was merciless with the dark hatred of desired revenge.

I knew I could not change the past. I could never have good parents, and they could never have a daughter who loved them while they were alive. Over time I worked on these things in my mind. I tried to put myself "in their shoes," as the saying goes.

It is difficult to forgive when two of the three people you are trying to reconcile with are dead, and you are married to the third. It also isn't easy to forgive yourself.

I started with Ma. The same coworker who pointed out to me that I was an abortion survivor helped me start down the road to forgiveness. He said, "She didn't try to kill *you*." Although the baby she wanted to kill was me, it wasn't like she had been taking care of me or talking to me or teaching me how to sit up or walk or developing a relationship with me. I was in her womb, and she had never seen me. That thought made me go back to what she had said to me once.

In the hospital, she had held me in her arms and told me

that she wanted to make a beautiful home for me. Maybe at some level, she knew what a mistake killing me would have been. Maybe she felt real sorrow for her actions.

I tried to understand how Ma must have felt when she realized she had given up her home in Bristol for a man who cheated on her. I tried to understand what Ma was thinking when she didn't take care of me, and when she told me she had tried to kill me. I tried to understand why Ma acted so mean and was so abusive. And, mostly, I tried to understand how she must have felt when I did or said things to let her know I not only didn't care for her, I actually had, at best, no emotions towards her. That last was the most painful and difficult for me.

Then I went through the same process with Pa. The thing I kept coming back to was the adultery. How could he not care what he did to his family? I came to the conclusion that he must have been a sex addict. Just because this is a relatively new term doesn't mean it isn't a condition that has existed forever. The man was willing to abuse his wife and neglect his daughter, and leave his home, for the sake of being intimate with other women. It really hurt me to come to the conclusion that sexual pleasure must have been more important to Pa than people, especially since I was one of those people. I understood that addiction was probably the issue, and that helped me understand Pa's actions. But try as I might, I could not read about sexual addiction. It disgusted and repelled me.

Pa was a slave to his passions; literally, he was not a free man. Nor was Ma free either, bound by her hatred and desire for revenge. And ultimately, I wasn't free. I was enslaved by my negative thoughts and actions, and my lack of forgiveness for Ma and Pa, and their thoughts and actions.

And lastly there was Jimmy. I felt devastated when he made me choose between him, and Ma and Pa, between security and no security. He forced this terrible choice on me, the woman he promised to love and cherish for life. I can now say I understand that very few people in the world could live in the squalor, or with the hostility, that was in that house. I could accept it because I had been raised in a filthy and bizarre house. I knew nothing else. Jimmy finally decided he couldn't take it anymore, and that I would have to choose between him and them. My accepting the reason behind the choice he insisted I make made it easier for me to forgive him.

I tried to understand the situations Ma, Pa, and Jimmy were in as they passed through life, and the dynamics of each situation. I also tried to understand why I interacted with these people, in particular situations, the way I did. I know we are all human and do things to others that we need to be forgiven for. Understanding why a person acted a certain way helped me heal. Ma and Pa were born in, and lived in, a different time than mine. Social roles and mores, rules of engagement, and repercussions for actions, were all different for them, born in the early 1900s, than for me, born in 1950. Ma and Pa lived through World War I and the Great Depression, through speakeasies and the era of flappers, black and white movies, and horses walking the streets before automobiles became popular. I have no idea what it would be like to live in those times.

So too for Jimmy, born fifteen years before me. He grew up with the effects of World War II and the threat of the Korean War. His time included radio shows, and black and white television, the beginning of color movies. He was young in the 1950s, the golden age of the family, when I was just learning how to sit up, walk, and talk. Or according to Pa, run and scream "fishbath." The four of us came from different times, and although we were all Americans, the America we knew was very different to each of us.

Ma, Pa, and Jimmy grew up in times in which women were not equal to men. It was expected that women would marry and have children, stay at home, and obey their husband. I suspect part of the marital relationship was not to inquire too closely into what a husband did before he came home late from work.

When I was born, life was still like that. I remember being told the worst fate a woman could face was being a spinster. Change in thinking started in my time. Women can now decide what they want to do with their lives – remain single, marry, work, travel, invest money, own property. It is in the ability to make decisions that I see equality, not in a false competition with men for power. And now, women in this country and in many others, have legal equality and protection under the law. Old attitudes and situations remain, but change continues.

I also had to learn to forgive myself. As I wrote in my Author's Note,

"In 1949, my mother tried to chemically abort me, and when I was eleven years old, she told me the story of that attempt. For many years afterward, I reacted to that information by making many of the same mistakes Ma and Pa had made, although to a greater degree. When I engaged in what I now realize was self-destructive behavior, I thought I was being independent, revolutionary, and avant-garde. When I started to look back at that time of my life, however, I could see my behavior seemed as if I had become a mutant hybrid of the worst of Ma and Pa together."

To be a good memoirist, a person must reveal, at a minimum, some representative examples of bad behavior. My actions mimicked Ma and Pa's behavior but became more serious, or stupid, than their actions. I acted like a Wild Child as a teenager.

I indiscriminately hated people. I hated Ma and Pa, their families, our neighbors, my teachers, even store clerks and policemen. Ma and Pa taught me how to hate. They hated a range of people – African Americans, almost all foreigners (especially "lace curtain Irish"), the wealthy, the poor, and in

Ma's case, all of Pa's girlfriends. Eventually, I came to realize that I didn't hate all people, but only those who had authority over me; perhaps because Ma and Pa had wielded their authority in an unjust manner.

In my fifties, I was stopped by a policeman for going through a red light. The car in front of me had slowed down after I entered the intersection, and I decided it would be better for me to continue to the other side rather than block traffic. I saw the policeman sitting in his cruiser by the side of the road, but I went through the light because I thought I had no choice.

He stopped me and told me I went through a red light. I told him I knew I had, and that I also knew that he saw I didn't have a choice. He asked for my license and registration, and I told him I was going to go into my pocketbook for my license and into my glove compartment for my registration. I took off my seat belt to reach both, and the policeman said, "Whoa, you were driving without a seat belt." I told him I knew he saw me take the seat belt off.

He gave me a ticket. I fought the ticket in traffic court. The fine was small, but I refused to tolerate his unjust use of authority. I won, but as I left, the policeman who signed me out said, "Just because you got off doesn't mean we believe you." Words said unjustly by a policeman in authority proved my point to me.

Today I do not have trouble with just authority. But to this day, I have trouble with the unjust use of authority, which I believe in this country is still rampant.

I lied, and I stole. I did those things to get people to do what I wanted them to do, or to give me what I wanted them to give me. I borrowed things and didn't return them, shoplifted, and stole money from Ma's crazy aunt. I acted this way because I had learned in Ma and Pa's house that any rule can be broken. Pa cheated on Ma, and Ma screamed at Pa, and they both neglected me. They had tried to kill me. The rules against adultery, spousal abuse, parental neglect, and murder were, I thought, important. And yet I saw those rules broken consistently.

I smoked pot and took uppers and downers. In the 1960s, these were common drugs available to the young. But I quickly realized my drug of choice was alcohol: white wine, sour mash whiskey, bourbon, and scotch. So, I switched from illegal drugs to legal ones. I liked those drinks fresh out of the bottle, no ice necessary. Over time, I must have drunk at least one vat of each.

Fortunately, one day I went to insert my key in a lock, and I couldn't do it because my hand was shaking so violently. I thought, *"Oh no! I have turned into Ma and Pa."* I immediately stopped drinking (many decades ago) and haven't touched a drop of liquor since then except for a pina colada after Jimmy's wake and a glass of white wine after his funeral.

I had boyfriends that I was too friendly with before I

married. I am ashamed to say that I do not remember their names. One day I thought, *"Oh no! I have turned into Pa."* So, I came to my senses and stopped having boyfriends.

When I married, and without my devout Catholic husband's knowledge, I continued to prevent pregnancy by using birth control pills, which gave me a blood clot, and then by using an IUD, which caused internal bleeding. Those two health issues made me realize I had to stop using birth control.

In hindsight, it does not surprise me that I did the foolish – and evil - things I did. Ma and Pa gave me plenty of examples of hatred, breaking rules, getting intoxicated, and in Pa's case, having illicit sex. On the other hand, even before Ma and Pa died, I had turned my life around, moving beyond their stilted worldview. I married and had a family; I earned several degrees and had a career.

Externally, I was a successful woman. But internally, I had bitter memories and my lack of forgiveness for Ma and Pa made those memories difficult to overcome.

One of the two things I regret the most, and have the most trouble forgiving myself for doing, is having boyfriends with whom I was too friendly. In fairness to me, I did not have any idea that in that kind of friendship, both people are lying with their bodies. John Paul II did not become pope until 1978, nor had he yet explained his deep thoughts on the theology of the body and lying with the body. I would not have listened to him when I was young anyway because I was not yet Catholic.

The second thing that I regret is using artificial means of birth control without my husband Jimmy's knowledge. He was a devout Catholic and never would have allowed such behavior. Decades after I stopped my bad behavior, and had become Catholic, I was sitting in a bioethics class when the professor, a Roman Catholic monsignor, stated that both birth control pills and IUDs do not merely prevent pregnancy. He said both cause spontaneous abortions. I was horrified!

A quick tabulation of how long I had used both forms of contraception led me to believe I could have been pregnant 30 or more times. I knew that a fertile woman could become pregnant each month and spontaneously abort, and in a month or two become pregnant again and spontaneously abort. And that means I could have 30 or more deceased children with my husband from the years I used birth control without his knowledge. That weighs heavily on my mind. My only hope is that if I attain heaven, I will meet those children there.

It took me a long time to process all that information – the things my parents had done to me and others, the mistakes I made, and the fact of the availability of immediate forgiveness.

I learned forgiveness, and I know that if I had not become Catholic, I never could have gotten to that point. Being Catholic made me understand. I realized I needed to resolve the issues in my life, but not to forget them. The past cannot be changed for me any more than for Ma and Pa and Jimmy. I cannot want revenge, nor justice in the "eye for an eye, tooth for a tooth" sense. To do so would continue to enslave me to memories, to resentment, and deep in my soul, at some level, to revenge. And it would mean that I would have to subject myself to the same standards. I cannot condone or excuse my behavior, nor the behavior of those three people.

But I can resolve it within myself. I can find integrity in my life while I seek a new relationship with my deceased Ma and Pa, my now deceased husband, Jimmy, and my deceased children that were sacrificed by means of birth control. I pray for them and ask them to pray for me.

Peace. I wanted peace. It has taken me years to move from a state of non-war to a state of peace. I would never have had that peace if Christ hadn't opened the door for me in the catacombs.

Epilogue

When I had almost completed the draft of this memoir, in 2015, my uncle's granddaughter, Ally, emailed me to tell me she had found eight letters from Pa to her father. Our two fathers had been close to each other. Ally's father had attended Pa's funeral and returned home to Boston. Apparently upset about Pa's death, he had gone out to a tavern, and when leaving, was killed by a drunk driver. The driver did not stop to help him. One of Ally's relatives had given her a bag of family letters after her father died in 1984. She had stored them in her cellar until she had an opportunity to go through them.

That night I called her, and for over three hours she read each of the letters to me, proceeding from the oldest to the newest. It was a difficult night for me, but I learned many things about Pa that I had never known. I think it was a difficult night for her too.

These are the things I learned.

Pa was a fairly educated man. His letters were well written, grammatically correct, and in a good amount of detail. He knew how to express himself well. This surprised me for two reasons. When I was a child, both Ma and Pa told me they had been taken out of school by their parents when they were young. Both of them told me they had never finished grammar school.

Because of what they said, I assumed that neither of them had much of an education. And later, when I was in college, I had Pa read my papers to see if there was anything that he thought should be changed. At one point, he told me he could not read my papers anymore because I had gone beyond what he was able to critique.

I was so surprised at how well Pa expressed himself that I looked both of them up in the 1940 Federal Decennial Census, which contained a column concerning education. Pa went through the second year of high school, and Ma through the third. I was stunned. How could they have come so close to graduating from high school but have both been pulled out of school by their parents? And why did they both tell me that it had occurred in grammar school?

Something else in Pa's letters surprised me. One of his cousins had offered to send him to Yale because he was so smart, but Pa's father didn't much care for that idea and said "no." Clearly, Pa could not have gone to Yale: a person has to be a high school graduate, come from a good background and have money to go to an Ivy League school. But perhaps his cousin would have sent him to a decent college.

Today I can no longer think of Ma and Pa as uneducated. They had at least some high school, which was quite an accomplishment in their time. I was born poor white trash, because they never used their education.

The second thing I learned from the letters was that Pa cared about me, at least to some extent. He said that when I was young, I had terrible allergies, all of which bothered my asthma. So, Pa worked to make sure I could go to a specialist every week, and Ma and I could take a cab to and from the doctor. He said in those days a doctor's visit cost two or three dollars, but the specialist cost twenty dollars.

What he wrote next was hard for me to hear. He said something to the effect of, "It was worth it because look at her now. She can walk, run, and jump." These were skills I needed as a retail security guard and an auxiliary policewoman, my jobs at the time the letters were written. Pa then wrote something funny. He couldn't understand how the auxiliary police could not know that I couldn't swim. He suspected I was afraid of water. He was correct. I am gut-wrenchingly terrified of being in the water.

The third thing I learned was that Pa was proud of me. He bragged about how I was in graduate school and how I went to conventions to give presentations.

I learned in several sentences that he didn't much care for Jimmy, which was okay because from my perspective the feeling was mutual. And he really wanted to go to Nova Scotia before he died.

Then I learned how he was baffled by Ma. She was always in and out of the hospital. In one letter, he said he couldn't understand why Ma didn't want him to visit her. This statement shocked me because I knew why she didn't want him around. She could never get over the adultery, and yet this didn't come to his mind. I could not understand this at all.

That question, and some other things he said about their life together before I was born gave me some insight into their relationship. He wrote at great length about how he and Ma had spent every weekend with Ma's relatives, Frank and Joan, and that they were inseparable friends. They would go drinking and dancing together. Neither Frank nor Ma liked to dance, but Pa and Joan did. He recalled how one night they were all out drinking. He and Joan danced to a drum solo. When the solo ended, they looked up, and no one else was on the dance floor. Everyone was standing around on the sides of the dance floor, watching them. I guess Ma and Pa liked to go out, or maybe she went to keep an eye on him, and he didn't know it.

The last thing I learned I found really heartbreaking. After Ma had died, Pa wrote that it was hell to get rid of her things and that he couldn't believe she was gone. Clearly, he felt sad at his loss.

Pa was educated, he liked and respected me, he couldn't understand why Ma didn't want him around, and he was sad that she had died. I feel heartbroken that I didn't know any of these things, and that he never expressed any of them to me.

If I had read those letters in 1984, perhaps I would have

started on the road to forgiveness earlier than I did. But then I would not have learned the true meaning – the supernatural truth – of forgiveness in our lives.

Made in the USA
Columbia, SC
10 July 2021